O G P L
OXFORD GENERAL PRACTICE LIBRARY

Musculoskeletal Problems

O G P L
OXFORD GENERAL PRACTICE LIBRARY

Musculoskeletal Problems

Dr Richard Davies

General Practitioner,
Cookridge, Leeds, UK

Dr Hazel Everitt

Research Training Fellow,
Department of Primary Care,
University of Southampton School of Medicine,
UK

Dr Chantal Simon

MRC Research Fellow and General Practitioner,
University of Southampton and Christchurch,
UK

and Series Editor

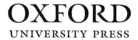

OXFORD
UNIVERSITY PRESS

OXFORD
UNIVERSITY PRESS

Great Clarendon Street, Oxford OX2 6DP

Oxford University Press is a department of the University of Oxford.
It furthers the University's objective of excellence in research, scholarship,
and education by publishing worldwide in

Oxford New York

Auckland Cape Town Dar es Salaam Hong Kong Karachi
Kuala Lumpur Madrid Melbourne Mexico City Nairobi
New Delhi Shanghai Taipei Toronto

With offices in

Argentina Austria Brazil Chile Czech Republic France Greece
Guatemala Hungary Italy Japan Poland Portugal Singapore
South Korea Switzerland Thailand Turkey Ukraine Vietnam

Oxford is a registered trade mark of Oxford University Press
in the UK and in certain other countries

Published in the United States
by Oxford University Press Inc., New York

British Library Cataloguing in Publication Data
Data available

Library of Congress Cataloguing in Publication Data
Data available

Typeset by Newgen Imaging Systems (P) Ltd, Chennai, India
Printed in Italy
on acid-free paper by
Legoprint S.p.A

ISBN 0–19–857058–9   978–0–19–857058–5

10 9 8 7 6 5 4 3 2 1

Contents

Acknowledgements

This book would not have come into being without the support and drive of Catherine Barnes, Georgia Pinteau and Sara Chare at Oxford University Press.

The material I was given to work with from the Oxford Handbook of General Practice, written by Hazel Everitt and Chantal Simon was outstanding to start with. I hope I have succeeded in improving it still further for this volume with the help and guidance of volume and series editor, Dr Chantal Simon.

I would also like to thank Dr Gavin Clunie, Mr David Hargreaves, Dr Francoise van Dorp and Mrs Lesley Boyd for their help with providing material for and reviewing this book, Dr Helen Lester for her help updating the changes to the Quality and Outcomes Framework, and Dr Anna Wilson for information and advice for the section on child protections issues.

Finally, all those who have ever written a book will know that the real burden is carried by those closest to the authors. I would like to thank my wife, Dr Ruth Davies, not only for her patience and support but also her clinical advice throughout.

RLD January 2006

Symbols and abbreviations

⚠	Warning
❶	Important Note
☙	Controversial point
☎	Telephone number
🖫	Website
▥	Cross reference to
±	With or without
↑	Increased/increasing
↓	Decreased/decreasing
→	Leading to
1°	Primary
2°	Secondary
♂	Male
♀	Female
≈	Approximately equal
~	Approximately
%	Percent(age)
≥	Greater than or equal to
≤	Less than or equal to
>	Greater than
<	Less than
+ve	Positive
−ve	Negative
°	Degrees
£	GMS contract payment available
C	Cochrane review
G	Guideline from major guideline producing body
N	NICE guidance
R	Randomized controlled trial in major journal
S	Systematic review in major journal
AA	Attendance Allowance
A&E	Accident and Emergency
AC	Acromioclavicular

AED	Automated external defibrillator
AIDS	Acquired immune deficiency syndrome
Alk phos	Alkaline phosphatase
ALS	Advance life support
ALT	Alanine-amino transferase
ANA	Anti-nuclear antibody
AS	Ankylosing spondylitis
AST	Asparatate amino transferase
bd	Twice daily
BLS	Basic life support
BMD	Bone mineral density
BMI	Body mass index
BMJ	British Medical Journal
BNF	British National Formulary
BP	Blood pressure
C	Cervical nerve root
Ca^{2+}	Calcium
CBT	Cognitive behaviour therapy
CCF	Congestive cardiac failure
CDH	Congenital dislocation of the hip
CFS	Chronic fatigue syndrome
CK	Creatine kinase
cm	Centimetre(s)
CMV	Cytomegalovirus
CNS	Central nervous system
CO_2	Carbon dioxide
COPD	Chronic obstructive pulmonary disease
COX2	Cyclo-oxygenase type 2
CPR	Cardiopulmonary resuscitation
Cr	Creatinine
CRP	C-reactive protein
CSF	Cerebrospinal fluid
CSM	Committee of Safety in Medicine
CVA	Stroke
CXR	Chest x-ray
d.	Day(s)
DEXA	Dual energy x-ray absorptionometry
DIP	Distal interphalyngeal
DLA	Disability Living Allowance

DM	Diabetes mellitus
DMARD	Disease modifying drug
DN	District nurse
DVLA	Driver and Vehicle Licensing Authority
DVT	Deep vein thrombosis
EBV	Epstein Barr virus
EC	Enteric coated
ECG	Electrocardiograph
e.g.	For example
ENT	Ear, nose and throat
ESR	Erythrocyte sedimentation rate
etc.	Et cetera
FBC	Full blood count
FH	Family history
g	gram (s)
GA	General anaesthetic
GCA	Giant cell arteritis
GI	Gastrointestinal
GMS	General Medical Services
GP	General Practitioner
GU	Genito-urinary
GUM	Gentio-urinary medicine
h.	Hour(s)
Hb	Haemoglobin
HRT	Hormone replacement therapy
HIV	Human immune deficiency virus
HV	Health visitor
IM	Intramuscular
IV	Intravenous
JCA	Juvenile chronic arthritis
JVP	Jugular venous pressure
K^+	Potassium
kg	Kilogram(s)
L	Lumbar nerve root
LA	Local anaesthetic
LFTs	Liver function tests
LMN	Lower motor neurone
LOC	Loss of consciousness
MAOI	Monoamine oxidase inhibitor

M,C&S	Microscopy, culture and sensitivities
MCP	Metacarpophalyngeal
MCV	Mean cell volume
mg	Milligrams
MI	Myocardial infarct
min.	Minutes
ml	Millitre(s)
MND	Motor neurone disease
mo.	Month(s)
MoD	Ministry of Defence
MRI	Magnetic resonance imaging
MS	Multiple sclerosis
MSU	Mid-stream urine
MTP	Metatarsophalyngeal
Na^+	Sodium
NHS	National Health Service
NICE	National Institute for Clinical Excellence
NSAID	Non-steroidal anti-inflammatory drug
O_2	Oxygen
OA	Osteoarthritis
od	Once daily
OT	Occupational therapy/therapist
OTC	Over the counter
OUP	Oxford University Press
oz	Ounce(s)
p.	Page number
PAN	Polyarteritis nodosa
PCO	Primary Care Organization
PD	Parkinson's disease
PE	Pulmonary embolus
Physio	Physiotherapy
PIP	Proximal interphalyngeal
PMH	Past medical history
PMR	Polymyalgia rheumatica
PMS	Personal Medical Services
PO_4	Phosphate
polio	Poliomyelitis
PPI	Proton pump inhibitor
prn	As needed

PTH	Parathyroid hormone
R	Right
RA	Rheumatoid arthritis
RhF	Rheumatoid factor
RSI	Repetitive strain injury
RTA	Road traffic accident
S	Sacral nerve root
s.	Second(s)
SI	Sacroiliac
SIGN	Scottish Intercollegiate Guidelines Network
SLE	Systemic lupus erythematosis
SLR	Straight leg raise
SSRI	Selective serotonin reuptake inhibitor
T	Thoracic nerve root
TB	Tuberculosis
TCA	Tricyclic antidepressant
tds	Three times a day
TENS	Transcutaneous electrical nerve stimulation
TFTs	Thyroid function tests
TIA	Transient ischaemic attack
u.	Units
UK	Uniter Kingdom
U&E	Urea and electrolytes
USS	Ultrascound scan
UTI	Urinary tract infection
WBC	White blood cell
WCC	White cell count
wk.	Week(s)
y.	Year(s)

Chapter 1

Assessing patients with musculoskeletal problems in primary care

1

Musculoskeletal assessment

When assessing a patient with musculoskeletal problems in primary care, the objectives are to:
- Establish a constructive relationship with the patient to enable patient and doctor to communicate effectively and serve as the basis for any subsequent therapeutic relationship.
- Determine whether the patient has a musculoskeletal problem and, if so, what that is.
- Find out (where possible) what caused that problem.
- Assess the patient's emotions and attitudes towards the problem.
- Establish how it might be treated.

History: Use open questions at the start, becoming directive when necessary – clarify, reflect, facilitate, listen. *Ask about:*

Presenting complaint: – Chronological account, past history of similar symptoms. Ask directly about:
- *Pain:* Pain is always subjective so take it at face value in *all* patients. Figure 1.1
- *Stiffness:* Where? How long? Present all the time or worse at certain times of day? Exacerbating and relieving factors
- *Deformity:* Swelling? If so, localized or diffuse? Bony deformity?
- *Loss of function:* e.g. locking, giving way, restriction in range of movement or pain making tasks impossible e.g. brushing hair, putting on socks, going up stairs
- *Previous treatments tried and result*

Occupation: Employed? Does the problem affect the job? Could the problem have been caused as a result of work?

Home situation: Housing, social support etc.

Family history: Rheumatology problems e.g. RA, OA

Attitudes and beliefs: How does the patient see the problem? What does he/she think is wrong? How does he/she think other people view the situation? What does the patient want you to do about it?

Examination: 📖 p.4

Action
- Summarize the history back to the patient and give an opportunity for the patient to fill in any gaps.
- Draw up a problem list and outline a management plan with the patient. Further investigations and interventions are guided by the findings on history and examination – so a good history and examination are essential.
- Set a review date.

Figure 1.1 Points to consider when taking a history of pain

S **Site of pain**: Where? Any radiation? Numbness where pain felt? Pattern of joint/muscle involvement?

O **Onset**: When did it start? How did it start? What started it? Change over time? History of injury?

C **Character of pain**: Type of pain – burning, shooting, stabbing, dull etc.

R **Radiation**: Does the pain go anywhere else?

A **Associated features**

T **Timing/pattern**: Is it worse at any time of day? Is it associated with any particular activities?

E **Exacerbating and relieving factors**

S **Severity**: Record especially if the pain is chronic and you want to measure change over time. Consider a patient diary. Ask about:
- Pain intensity e.g. none–mild–moderate–severe; rank on a 1–10 scale.
- Record interference with sleep or usual activities
- Pain relief e.g. none–slight–moderate–good–complete

GP Notes: Useful screening questions

- Do you have any pain or stiffness in your muscles, joints or back?
- Can you dress yourself completely without any difficulty?
- Can you walk up and down stairs without any difficulty?

⚠ Be aware of 2° gain from pain if symptoms seem out of proportion – outstanding compensation claims are a significant factor in success of pain management.

General rules for examination

General inspection: Watch the patient throughout the consultation:
- How did he walk into the room?
- Does he use a walking aid or any other aid or appliance?
- Is there any obvious deformity?
- Is his posture normal?
- How does he get onto the examination couch?
- Is he in obvious discomfort or distress?

General rules for musculoskeletal examination: Figure 1.2
Specific examination:
- Hands and wrists 📖 p.88
- Elbows 📖 p.86
- Shoulder 📖 p.80
- Neck 📖 p.70
- Back 📖 p.74
- Hips 📖 p.96
- Knees 📖 p.102
- Ankles and feet 📖 p.110

Neurology: Think systematically about the level of neurological lesions associated with musculoskeletal problems. *Potential sites:* muscle; neuromuscular junction; along the course of the nerve outside the spinal cord; within the spinal cord; and within the brain. ❶ Remember >1 nerve may be affected by a single lesion and neurological problems may result in musculoskeletal abnormalities. *Check:*
- *Posture*
- *Muscle bulk:* muscle wasting? muscle hypertrophy?
- *Abnormal movements:* fasciculation? involuntary movements? compensatory movements?
- *Tone:* ↑, normal or ↓
- *Power:* test movements in the affected area – Table 1.1, 📖 p.6
- *Reflexes:* see below
- *Co-ordination:* finger–nose test; heel-along-shin test; rapid alternating movements
- *Sensation:* light touch, pin prick, cold, vibration, joint position sense (especially distally) – Figures 1.3 and 1.4, 📖 pp.8–9

Reflexes: Automatic responses. The reflex arc goes from the stimulus via a sensory nerve to the spinal cord and then back along a motor nerve to cause muscle contraction, without brain involvement.
Key tendon reflexes: Table 1.3, 📖 p.7
- *Absent or ↓reflex:* Implies a breach in the reflex arc at:
  - Sensory nerve or root e.g. neuropathy, spondylosis
  - Anterior horn cell e.g. MND, polio
  - Motor nerve or root e.g. neuropathy, spondylosis
  - Nerve endings e.g. myasthenia gravis, *or*
  - Muscle e.g. myopathy
- *↑reflex:* Implies lack of higher control – an upper motor neurone lesion e.g. post-stroke

Clonus: Rhythmic involuntary muscle contraction due to abrupt tendon stretching e.g. by dorsiflexing the ankle – associated with an UMN lesion.

Common mononeuropathies: Table 1.2, 📖 p.6

Figure 1.2 General rules for musculoskeletal examination

Look
- Compare right with left.
- Check skin for erythema, scars and rashes e.g. psoriasis vasculitis.
- Check for swelling and possible effusions.
- Check for hypertrophy and inflammation of synovium (RA).
- Check for bony outgrowths (OA).
- Deformity suggests chronic destructive arthritis (e.g. RA) or previous trauma.
- Look for subluxation and dislocation.
- Check for muscle wasting.

Feel
- Assess temperature of joints with back of fingers – warn joints may indicate synoviotis, infection or crystal arthritis.
- Tenderness – What is the exact structure which is tender? Is there a pattern of disease?
- Palpate swellings – distinguish the soft swelling of synovitis from fluctuant swellings of effusions and hard, immobile bony swellings.

Move
- Passive movement is used to assess the joint itself – ask the patient to relax the limb and allow the examiner to move the joint.
- Active movement demonstrates function e.g. hand function, gait.
- Abnormal movements – assess joint stability by trying to move the joint in abnormal directions.
- Joint crepitus indicates irregularity of articular surfaces and suggests a chronic problem.

Measure
- Record an estimate of range of movement (e.g. straight leg raise). Range of movement can be measured more accurately with a goniometer (a hinged rod with a central protractor) if available.
- A tape measure can help monitor serial muscle bulk.

Table 1.1 Quick screening tests for muscle power

Joint	Movement	Nerve roots	Joint	Movement	Nerve roots
Shoulder	Abduction Adduction	C5,6 C6–8	Hip	Flexion Extension	L1–3 L4,5 & S1
Elbow	Flexion Extension	C5,6 C7,8	Knee	Flexion Extension	L5 & S1 L3,4
Wrist	Flexion Extension	C7,8 C6,7	Ankle	Dorsiflexion Plantarflexion	L4,5 S1,2
Fingers	Flexion Extension Abduction	C8,T1 C7,8 T1	Toes	Extensors Flexors	L5,S1 S2

Test proximal muscle power by asking the patient to sit from lying, pull you towards him/herself or rise from squatting.

Table 1.2 Common mononeuropathies

Nerve involved	Nerve roots	Presentation	Common causes
Median	C5–T1	Loss of sensation over lateral 3½ fingers and palm. Wasting of the thenar eminence. Inability to flex the terminal phalanx of the thumb implies involvement of the anterior interosseous branch.	Trauma (especially wrist lacerations), carpal tunnel syndrome
Ulnar	C7–T1	Weakness and wasting of interossei muscles (weakness of abduction of fingers) and claw hand deformity, wasting of hypothenar eminence, sensory loss over medial 1½ fingers and ulnar side of the hand. Flexion of 4th and 5th fingers is weak if the lesion is proximal.	Trauma or compression at the elbow, trauma at the wrist
Radial	C5–T1	Sensory loss is variable but always includes the dorsal aspect of the root of the thumb. Wrist drop and weak extension of thumb and fingers.	Compression against the humerus, trauma
Sciatic	L4–S2	Weakness of hamstrings and all muscles below the knee (foot drop), loss of sensation below the knee laterally.	Back injury, pelvic tumours
Common peroneal	L4–S2	Inability to dorsiflex the foot (foot drop), evert the foot, extend the toes. Sensory loss over dorsum of the foot.	Trauma
Tibial	S1–S3	Inability to stand on tiptoe, invert the foot or flex toes. Sensory loss over sole.	Trauma or entrapment

Table 1.3 Reflexes and nerve roots involved: record whether absent, present with reinforcement, normal or brisk ± clonus

Reflex	Test	Expected result	Nerve roots
Biceps	Tap a finger placed on the biceps tendon by letting the tendon hammer fall on it	Contraction of the biceps + elbow flexion	C5, C6
Supinator	Tap the lower end of the radius just above the wrist with the tendon hammer	Contraction of brachioradialis + elbow flexion	C5,C6
Triceps	Support elbow in flexion with 1 hand. Tap the triceps tendon with a tendon hammer held in the other hand	Contraction of the triceps + elbow extension	C7,C8
Knee	Support the knees so relaxed and slightly bent. Let the tendon hammer fall onto the infrapatellar tendon	Contraction of quadriceps + extension of the knee	L3,L4
Ankle	Externally rotate the thigh and flex the knee. Let the tendon hammer fall onto the Achilles tendon	Contraction of the gastrocnemius + plantar flexion of the ankle	S1
Abdominal	Lightly stroke the abdominal wall diagonally towards the umbilicus in each of the four abdominal quadrants	Abdominal wall contractions. When absent can be normal or indicate UMN or LMN lesion	T7–T12
Cremaster	♂ patients only. Pre-warn the patient. Stroke the superior and medial aspect of the thigh in a downwards direction	Contraction of the cremasteric muscle → raising of scrotum and testis on the side stroked. Absent in UMN and LMN lesions	L1
Anal	Scratch the perianal skin	Reflex contraction of the external sphincter. Absent in UMN and LMN lesions	S4,S5
Plantar	Pre-warn the patient. Run a blunt object up the lateral side of the sole of the foot, curving medially before the MTP joints	Flexion of the big toe (if >1y. old). Extension implies UMN lesion	S1

🛈 Reinforcement: Method of accentuating reflexes. Use if a reflex seems absent. Ask the patient to clench their teeth (to reinforce upper limb reflexes) or clench their hands and pull in opposite directions (to accentuate lower limb reflexes). This effect only lasts ~1s., so ask the patient to perform the manoeuvre simultaneously with the tap from the tendon hammer.

Figure 1.3 Dermatomes and peripheral nerve distribution

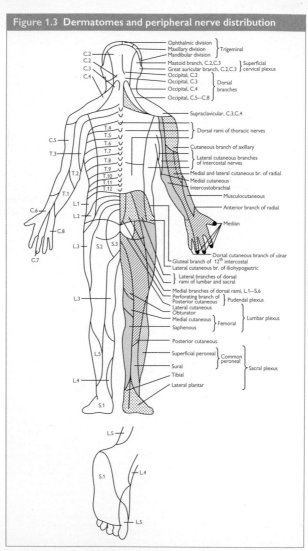

Figure 1.4 Dermatomes and peripheral nerve distribution

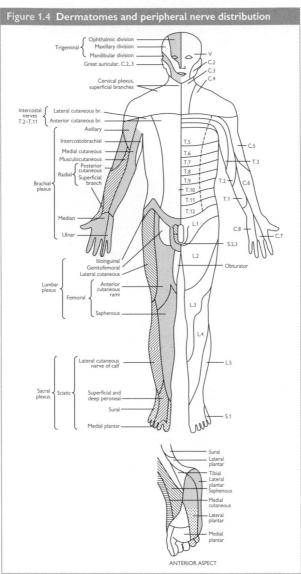

ANTERIOR ASPECT

Reproduced from Oxford Handbook of Clinical Medicine 6e, edited by Longmore & Wilkinson (2004). By permission of Oxford University Press.

Symptoms of common musculoskeletal disorders

Joint pain: Figure 1.5
Common arthropathies: 📖 pp.126–147

- Osteoarthritis
- Rheumatoid arthritis
- Ankylosing spondylitis
- SLE
- Reactive arthritis
- Psoriatic arthritis
- Enteropathic arthropathy
- Gout or pseudogout
- Sicca syndrome
- Malignancy

Bone pain: *Consider:*
- *Fracture:* due to injury, stress fracture or pathological fracture
- *Arthritis:* referred pain from affected joints
- *Malignancy:* primary bone malignancy, haematological malignancy e.g. multiple myeloma, or secondaries (usually from breast, prostate, lung, thyroid, kidney – more rarely bowel, melanoma)
- *Benign bone tumour*
- *Osteomyelitis*
- *Metabolic causes:* e.g. hypercalcaemia

Muscle pain/myalgia: Isolated myalgia can be a result of overuse or soft tissue injury. Generalized myalgia is associated with many diseases including:
- Infection
- Polymyalgia rheumatica (usually in shoulder/hip girdle distribution)
- Fibromyalgia
- Drugs e.g. statin use
- Rare diseases e.g. Wegener's granulomatosis, PAN

Cramp: Painful muscle spasm. Common – especially at night and after exercise. Rarely associated with disease – salt depletion, muscle ischaemia, myopathy. Forearm cramps suggest motor neurone disease. Night cramps in the elderly may respond to quinine sulphate 200mg nocte (may take 4wk to work-reassess every 3mo. for ongoing need).

Dystonia: Prolonged muscle contraction producing abnormal postures or repetitive movements.
- *Spasmodic torticollis:* head is pulled to one side and held there by a contracting sternomastoid muscle. Exclude infection as a cause. Treat with physiotherapy.
- *Blepharospasm:* involunary contraction of the orbicularis oculi.
- *Writer's cramp:* spasm of the hand and forearm muscles on writing.

Facial pain: Treat the cause. *Common causes include:* trigeminal neuralgia; temporomandibular joint disorders; dental disorders; sinusitis; migrainous neuralgia; shingles; and post-herpetic neuralgia.

No cause is found in many patients – it is then termed *atypical facial pain*. Atypical facial pain may respond to simple analgesia with paracetamol or a NSAID. If this fails, try nerve painkillers e.g. amitriptyline 25–75mg nocte. Refer those with troublesome symptoms to ENT or neurology .

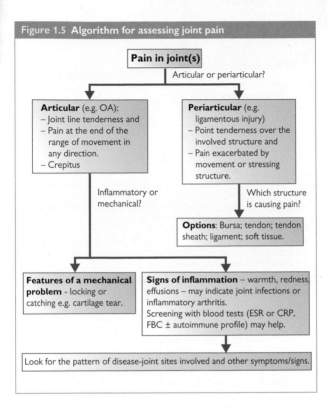

Figure 1.5 Algorithm for assessing joint pain

Pain in joint(s)

Articular or periarticular?

Articular (e.g. OA):
– Joint line tenderness and
– Pain at the end of the range of movement in any direction.
– Crepitus

Periarticular (e.g. ligamentous injury)
– Point tenderness over the involved structure and
– Pain exacerbated by movement or stressing structure.

Inflammatory or mechanical?

Which structure is causing pain?

Options: Bursa; tendon; tendon sheath; ligament; soft tissue.

Features of a mechanical problem - locking or catching e.g. cartilage tear.

Signs of inflammation – warmth, redness, effusions – may indicate joint infections or inflammatory arthritis.
Screening with blood tests (ESR or CRP, FBC ± autoimmune profile) may help.

Look for the pattern of disease-joint sites involved and other symptoms/signs.

11

GP Notes: ⚠ Red flags – features of joint pain which should prompt early/urgent referral

Single joint
• Inflamed joint with associated fever or constitutional disturbance – beware of infection.
• Any joint which is 'locked' or so painful that movement is impossible.
• Severe pain at rest or at night
• Pain that gets relentlessly worse over a period of days or weeks.

Multiple joints
• Severe systemic symptoms – high fevers, significant weight loss or a very ill patient (suggests rheumatoid arthritis, sepsis or malignancy)
• Focal systemic signs e.g. rashes, nodules or GI disturbances.
• Severe pain and/or inability to function.

Chest deformity

- *Barrel chest:* AP diameter ↑, expansion ↓. Seen with chronic hyperinflation (e.g. asthma/COPD).
- *Pigeon chest (pectus carinatum):* Prominent sternum with a flat chest. Seen in patients with chronic childhood asthma or rickets.
- *Funnel chest (pectus excavatum):* The lower end of sternum is depressed.
- *Harrison's sulcus:* Groove deformity of the lower ribs at the diaphragm attachment site. Suggests chronic childhood asthma or rickets.
- *Kyphosis:* ↑ forward spinal convexity. Usually affects the thoracic spine.
  - *Postural kyphosis* ('drooping shoulders' or 'roundback') is common and voluntarily correctable.
  - *Structural kyphosis* cannot be corrected voluntarily. *Common causes:* osteoporosis, Paget's disease, ankylosing spondylitis and adolescent kyphosis (Scheuermann's disease). May cause a restrictive ventilatory defect.
- *Scoliosis:* 📖 pp.20–1, 30–3, 74, 118.

Chest pain: Common symptom.

> ⚠ Always think: could this be an MI, PE, dissecting aneurysm or pericariditis?

History: Ask about site and nature of pain, duration, associated symptoms (e.g. breathlessness, nausea), provoking and relieving factors, PMH, drug history, smoking history, FH (e.g. heart disease).

Examination: Check BP in both arms, general appearance (distress, sweating, pallor), JVP, apex beat, heart sounds, lung fields, local tenderness, pain on movement of chest, skin rashes, swelling or tenderness of legs (?DVT).

Investigations: ECG and CXR may be helpful depending on history and examination.

Management: Treat the cause (Table 1.4).

Musculoskeletal chest pain is common. It can be a sharp or dull pain and is due to radiation of pain from the thoracic spine or local muscular or bone injury (e.g. fractured rib). It is usually made worse by movement and relieved by rest and/or NSAIDs. May be locally tender. Usually diagnosed on history alone and requires no investigation – except to exclude other causes of chest pain. Settles spontaneously.

Table 1.4 Causes of acute chest pain

Diagnosis	Features
MI	Band-like pain around the chest or central chest pressure/dull ache ± radiation to shoulders, arms (left > right), neck and/or jaw. Often associated with nausea, sweating and/or shortness of breath.
Unstable angina	As for MI.
Pericarditis	Sharp, constant sternal pain relieved by sitting forwards. May radiate to left shoulder ± arm or into the abdomen. Worse lying on the left side and on inspiration, swallowing and coughing.
Dissecting thoracic aneurysm	Typically presents with sudden tearing chest pain radiating to the back. Consider in any patient with chest pain (especially if radiates through to the back) and ↓BP.
PE	Acute dyspnoea, sharp chest pain (worse on inspiration), haemoptysis and/or syncope. Tachycardic and mild pyrexia.
Pleurisy	Sharp, localized chest pain, worse on inspiration. May be associated with symptoms and signs of a chest infection.
Pneumothorax	Sudden onset of pleuritic chest pain or ↑ breathlessness ± pallor and tachycardia.
Oesophageal spasm, oesophagitis	Central chest pain. May be associated with acid reflux (though not always). May be described as burning but often indistinguishable from cardiac pain. May respond to antacids.
Musculoskeletal pain	Localized pain – worse on movement. May be a history of injury.
Shingles	Intense, often sharp, unilateral pain. Responds poorly to analgesia. May be present several days before rash appears. Rash does not cross the midline.
Costochondritis	Inflammation of the costochondral junctions – tenderness over the costochondral junction and pain in the affected area on springing the chest wall.
Bornholm's disease	Unilateral chest and/or abdominal pain, rhinitis. Coxsackie virus infection. Treat with simple analgesia.
Idiopathic chest pain	No cause apparent. Common. Affects young people > elderly people. ♀ > ♂

13

GP Notes: Chest pain

⚠ If a patient is acutely unwell with chest pain and the cause is not clear, err on the side of caution and admit for further assessment.

Walking problems

Walking difficulty ('off legs'): Common amongst the elderly.
Causes:

- *Musculoskeletal:* Osteoarthritis or RA, osteoporotic fractures, fractured neck of femur, osteomalacia, Paget's disease, polymyalgia rheumatica
- *Psychological:* Depression, bereavement, fear of falling
- *Neurological:* Stroke, Parkinson's disease, peripheral neuropathy, subdural haematoma
- *Spinal cord compression*
- *Systemic:* Pneumonia, UTI, anaemia, hypothyroidism, renal failure, infection, hypothermia

Management: Treat according to cause. Refer if inadequate support at home, cause warrants admission or no cause is found.

Abnormal gait: Gait means manner of walking. Abnormal gait can give clues to the underlying problem.

Abnormal movements: Normal gait is interrupted by abnormal movements e.g. choreiform movements, athetoid movements or hemiballismus. May indicate underlying neurological problem e.g. cerebral palsy, Huntington's chorea.

Antalgic gait: Gait adjusts to try to minimize pain in a joint – usually OA hip. The patient leans towards the affected side and takes a rapid step on that side followed by a slower step on the contralateral side.

Drunken gait: As its name suggests, a drunken gait is the type of gait adopted by someone who is drunk. The other major cause is a cerebellar lesion. *Features:*

- Wide-based gait or reeling gait on a narrow base
- Feet are often raised too high and placed over carefully with the patient looking ahead
- If a cerebellar lesion, the patient falls to the side of the lesion

Foot drop: Patients have a high-stepping gait to prevent scraping the toe on the ground.

Frontal lesions: Marked unsteadiness – the feet appear stuck to the floor causing a wide-based, shuffling gait.

Hemiplegic gait: Style of walking seen in patients with UMN lesions. *Features:*

- Arm adducted and internally rotated, elbow flexed and pronated ± finger flexion
- Foot is plantar flexed and the leg swings in a lateral arc

Parkinsonian gait: Seen in patients with Parkinson's disease and other causes of Parkinsonism. *Features:*

- *Akinesia:* Hesitation in starting walking (may be relieved by placing a line on the floor for the patient to step over).
- *Marche au petit pas:* Small, shuffling steps.

- *Festinant gait:* Flexed posture as if hurrying to keep up with feet.
- Lack of normal arm swing.
- *Kinesia paradoxica:* Patients can perform fast or energetic movements more easily than slow ones e.g. running may be easier than walking.

Scissor gait: As the name implies, the patient walks as if their legs were like a pair of scissors. Associated with spastic paraplegia:
- Both legs are held rigid with plantar flexion of the ankle, extension of the knee and adduction/internal rotation of the hips.
- The patient walks on tiptoe and the knees rub together/cross during the walking cycle.
- Often accompanied by complex movements of the upper limbs to assist the walking movements.

Sensory ataxic gait: Loss of proprioception due to peripheral neuropathy or spinal cord disease (e.g. cervical spondylosis, MS, syphilis, combined degeneration of the cord) results in an ataxic gait similar to that seen with cerebellar disease. *Features:*
- Broad-based gait with a tendency to stamp feet down clumsily.
- Patient tends to look at feet throughout the walking cycle.
- Romberg's sign +ve.

Waddling gait: Typically seen in patients with proximal myopathy e.g. due to muscular dystrophy. Other causes: pregnancy, congenital dislocation of the hip hypothyroidism. *Features:*
- Broad-based gait in which the pelvis drops to the side of the leg being raised.
- The patient moves his body and hips to accommodate this, resulting in a duck-like waddle in the swing phase.
- Commonly accompanied by ↑ forward curvature of the lower spine.

Tired all the time

Tiredness is a common symptom of rheumatological conditions but almost any disease processes can cause tiredness – whether physical or psychological. Physical causes account for ~9% of cases; 75% have symptoms of emotional distress.

Fatigue is common. 1:400 sustained episodes of fatigue generate a GP consultation. GPs see 30 patients/y. whose main complaint is fatigue and it may be a secondary symptom in many others. 2% of consultations with fatigue result in secondary care referral.

Assessment: Figure 1.6

Common organic causes of fatigue in general practice
- Anaemia
- Infections (EBV, CMV, hepatitis)
- DM
- Hypo- or hyperthyroidism
- Perimenopausal
- Asthma
- Carcinomatosis
- Sleep apnoea
- Inflammatory conditions e.g. RA, PMR

Management:
- Treat organic causes.
- In most no physical cause is found – reassure.
- Explaining the relationship of psychological and emotional factors to fatigue can help patients deal with symptoms.
- If lasts >6–12wk and symptoms/signs of depression, consider a trial of antidepressants e.g. sertraline 50mg od.

Refer those with:
- Chronic or disabling fatigue with no identifiable cause
- Suspected sleep apnoea
- Suspected chronic fatigue syndrome
- If referral is requested by the patient

Figure 1.6 **Assessment of patients presenting with fatigue**

History:

Onset & duration – short history and abrupt onset suggest post-viral cause or onset of DM, protracted course suggests emotional origin

Pattern of fatigue – fatigue on exertion which goes away with rest suggests an organic cause whilst fatigue worst in the morning which never goes siggests depression.

Associated symptoms e.g. breathlessness, weight loss or anorexia suggest underlying organic disease. Chronic pain may cause fatigue.

Sleep patterns – early morning wakening and unrefreshing sleep may suggest depression, whilst snoring, pauses of breathing in sleep and sleepiness in the day time suggest sleep apnoea.

Psychiatric history – ask about depression, anxiety, stress; medication. Ask what the patient thinks is wrong and their underlying fears.

Examination: Full examination unless history suggests cause.
🚫 Most examinations will be normal.

Investigations:

Suitable initial investigations are: FBC, ESR, TFTs, blood glucose, U&E, LFTs, Ca^{2+}, monospot test, MSU for M,C&S. 🚫 Viral titres don't help.

Screening questionnaires for depression can be useful.

Further investigations (e.g. autoimmune profile) may be necessary depending on initial test results, clinical findings and course.

⚠ Don't over-investigate – 1:3 patients have ≥ 1 abnormal result in a standard battery of tests abnormal results are relevant to symptoms in <1:10 of those patients.

Screening for musculoskeletal problems in childhood

Congenital dislocation of the hip (CDH): Also referred to as developmental dysplasia of the hip (DDH). Encompasses varying degrees of instability, subluxation and dysplasia of the hip joint. Screening should take place at birth, at the 6wk. check, at 6–8mo. and in the second year (15–21mo.). High-risk children (breech babies, family history, foot deformities, sternomastoid tumour) are routinely screened with USS. Screening tests should be taught *in vivo* by someone experienced in the technique.

Screening a child <3mo.:
- In the newborn period limited abduction is uncommon as a sign of dislocation of the hip and more likely to be due to ↑ tone e.g. spina bifida. At this time the most important sign is instability of the hip.
- Screening tests should be performed in a warm room with the baby undressed and lying on a firm surface.
- Flex hips and knees to 90° using one hand for each leg with thumbs on the inner side of the baby's knee and ring and little fingers behind the greater trochanters (Figure 1.7).
- Each hip is tested separately. The examiner's hand on the opposite side from the hip being tested is used to stabilize the pelvis. Hold the thumb over the symphysis pubis and fingers under the sacrum.
- Only test once as repeated testing can damage the hips.

Ortolani manoeuvre: Each hip is gently abducted whilst lifting the greater trochanter forward. As a dislocated hip is abducted a clunk or jumping sensation is felt. It is difficult to tell the difference between a click of a normal hip and a clunk of an abnormal one – so refer any clicky or clunky hips for further investigation (usually USS or orthopaedic review).

Barlow manoeuvre: This establishes whether the hips are dislocatable. Holding the legs as described above, gently apply pressure along the line of the femur, pushing it backwards out of the acetabulum. The judder of the femoral head slipping in and out of the acetabulum can be felt if the hip is dislocatable.

Screening a child >3mo.:
- After 3mo. of age, limited abduction is the most common finding in children with CDH. If the infant lies on his back with hips flexed at 90°, any hip which cannot abduct >75° should be viewed with suspicion.
- Perform the Ortolani and Barlow tests.
- *Other signs:*
  - Limb shortening on the affected side – compare knee levels.
  - Asymmetry of the thighs – particularly skin creases.
  - Flattening of the buttock – in a prone position, the affected side may look flatter.

Figure 1.7 Screening for congenital dislocation of the hip (Ortolani test)

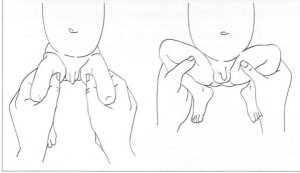

Diagram reproduced from Forfar & Arneil's Textbook of Pediatrics 6e, McIntosh, © 2003, with permission from Elsevier.

Screening for childhood scoliosis: Early treatment of scoliosis prevents progression. Early-onset scoliosis (<8y.) is responsible for cosmetic problems, pain and cardiopulmonary disturbance. Late-onset scoliosis is less severe but also causes pain and significant deformity.

Risk factors:
- Congenital malformations of the spine (butterfly vertebra)
- Neuromuscular problems e.g. cerebral palsy
- Connective tissue disorders
- Neurofibromatosis
- Bone dysplasias
- Friedrich's ataxia

Clinical features:
- Difference in shoulder height
- Spinal curvature
- Difference in space between trunk and upper limbs

🛈 Scoliosis which disappears on bending is postural and of no clinical significance.

Screening tests:
- **<1y. old:** Place the child prone on their tummy and feel the shoulder and thoracic cage. There should be no rib hump or shoulder hump.
- **>1y. old:** Ask the child to bend forward whilst standing straight with both feet together and holding both hands straight. Look for a shoulder, thoracic or lumbar hump, difference in shoulder height, and/or obvious spinal curvature (Figure 1.8). Check the gap between arm and waistline.

⚠ In all cases, if scoliosis is suspected, refer for an orthopaedic opinion.

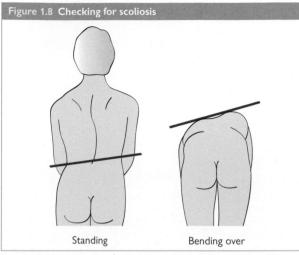

Figure 1.8 Checking for scoliosis

Standing   Bending over

Chapter 2

Diagnosis and management of common childhood musculoskeletal problems

Birth trauma

Head trauma

Caput succedaneum: Swelling, bruising and oedema of the presenting portion – usually scalp. Unsightly but resolves spontaneously.

Cephalhaematoma: Uncommon. Haemorrhage beneath the periosteum. Unilateral and usually parietal. Presents as a lump – the size of an egg – on the baby's head. Treatment is not required, but anaemia or hyperbilirubinaemia may follow.

Depressed skull fractures: Rare. Most result from forceps pressure; rarely caused by the head resting on a bony prominence *in utero*. May be associated with subdural bleeding, subarachnoid haemorrhage, or contusion/laceration of the brain itself. Seen and felt as a depression in the skull. X-ray confirms diagnosis; neurosurgical elevation may be needed.

Intracranial haemorrhage: Rare. Suggested by lack of responsiveness, fits, respiratory distress ± shock. Admit as an emergency.

Nerve injuries

Cranial nerve trauma: The facial nerve is injured, most often causing facial asymmetry, especially during crying. Usually resolves spontaneously by 2–3mo. of age. Refer to paediatric neurology if not resolving.

Brachial plexus injury: Follows stretching caused by shoulder dystocia, breech extraction, or hyperabduction of the neck in cephalic presentations. Often associated with other traumatic injuries e.g. fractured clavicle or humerus.
- *Partial injuries of the brachial plexus:* Most recover but site and type of nerve root injury determine the prognosis. If persistent >3mo., refer to paediatric neurology for further investigation. A biceps deficit lasting >3mo. has poor prognosis and requires surgery, Figure 2.1.
  - Injuries of the upper brachial plexus (C5–6) affect muscles around the shoulder and elbow – *Erb's palsy.*
  - Injuries of the lower plexus (C7–8 and T1) affect primarily muscles of the forearm and hand – *Klumpke's palsy.*
- *Injuries of the entire brachial plexus:* No movement of the arm + sensory loss. Refer immediately for neurological opinion. Prognosis for recovery is poor.

Fractures

Midclavicular fracture: Most common fracture during birth. Usually occurs due to shoulder dystocia. Refer if suspected. Most clavicular fractures are greenstick and heal rapidly and uneventfully. A large callus forms at the fracture site in <1wk. and remodelling is completed in <1mo. Can be associated with brachial plexus injury and/or pneumothorax.

Long bone fractures: The humerus and femur may be fractured during difficult deliveries. Refer if suspected. Usually long bones heal rapidly without any residual deformity.

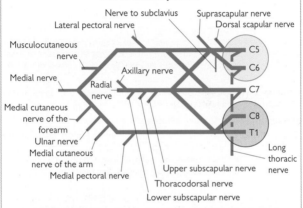

Figure 2.1 Brachial plexus injuries in neonates

Erb's palsy
Arm hangs limply by the side and looks like a waiter
asking for a tip, shoulder medially rotated, forearm
pronated and wrist flexed.
Loss of sensation on lateral aspect of arm.

The brachial plexus

Nerve to subclavius   Suprascapular nerve
Lateral pectoral nerve   Dorsal scapular nerve

Musculocutaneous
nerve   C5

            Axillary nerve   C6

Medial nerve
        Radial   C7
        nerve

Medial cutaneous
nerve of the   C8
forearm
Ulnar nerve   T1
Medial cutaneous   Long
nerve of the arm   thoracic
Medial pectoral nerve   Upper subscapular nerve   nerve
                    Thoracodorsal nerve
              Lower subscapular nerve

Klumpke's palsy
Paralysis of all the small muscles of the hand, causing clawing.
Loss of sensation along the medial aspect of the arm.
Rarely accompanied by Horner's syndrome.

Congenital orthopaedic problems

Major congenital abnormality occurs in ~1:50 babies. Many more have minor abnormalities.

Polydactyly and syndactyly

Polydactyly: Extra digits can vary from small fleshy tags to complete duplications. They may be an isolated defect or associated with syndromes. Small fleshy tags are removed in the first few months. For extra digits firmly fixed or involving tendons or joints, surgery is delayed until the child is >1y. bigger. Refer to orthopaedics or plastic surgery.

Syndactyly: Digits may be joined by a web of skin or more firmly fused. Webbing is usually mild and treatment is for cosmetic reasons, if at all. Where digits are fused separation and skin grafting is carried out at ~4y. Refer to plastic surgery.

Club foot (talipes): Consists of inversion of the foot, adduction of forefoot relative to hindfoot and equinus (plantar flexion).

Positional talipes: Moulding deformity seen in neonates. The foot can be passively everted and dorsiflexed to the normal position. Treatment is with physiotherapy. Follow up to check the deformity is resolving.

True talipes: The foot *cannot* be passively everted and dorsiflexed to the normal position. Refer to orthopaedics. Treatment is with physiotherapy, splints ± surgery.

Congenital dislocation of the hip (CDH): Also referred to as developmental dysplasia of the hip (DDH). 3:2000 live births (♀:♂ ≈ 6:1) – though 10x that number have unstable hips and even more have 'clicks' detected on routine neonatal screening. Often there is a family history of CDH. Associated with breech presentation at term.

Presentation
- Usually detected at routine neonatal screening 📖 p.18.
- High-risk infants (e.g. breech babies or those with family history of CDH) are additionally routinely screened with USS at 6wk. of age.
- Despite screening some cases slip though the net. They present as toddlers with limp/waddling gait; frequent falls; asymmetric thigh creases or limited hip adduction noted at later developmental checks.
- Rarely some go unnoticed until adulthood when they present with premature osteoarthritis.

Management: Refer to an orthopaedic surgeon specializing in paediatric problems. Treatment depends on when the condition is diagnosed:
- *Young babies:* Splinting in a pelvic harness to reduce and hold the hips – the hips are held in partial abduction using slings under each thigh attached to a body harness e.g. von Rosen splint. Usually babies wear a splint for ~3mo.
- *Older babies, toddlers and adults:* Surgery is required.

Congenital scoliosis: 📖 p.30

Advice for patients: Support for parents and children

• Steps Support for patients with lower limb conditions and their families: ☎ 0871 717 0044 🖳 www.steps-charity.org.uk

Hypermobility syndrome: Occurs in children or young adults with lax joints. <½ are symptomatic. Those that have symptoms present with recurrent joint pains – mainly affecting the knees. Other symptoms include joint effusion, dislocation, ligamentous injuries, low back pain and premature osteoarthritis. The condition is benign, and joints become stiffer with age. Treatment, when needed, is with physiotherapy. Rarely associated with rare congenital disorders e.g. Ehlers-Danlos syndrome.

Neural tube defects: Most neural tube defects are detected ante-natally at routine antenatal screening. Types of defect:

- *Anencephaly:* Absent cerebral cortex and skull vault. Incompatible with life – those infants born alive die within hours of birth.
- *Cranium defects:* Vary in severity from meningocoele (meninges protrude through the defect) to inoperable encephalocoele (brain tissue protrudes through skull).
- *Spina bifida:* The vertebral arch is incomplete.
  - *Occulta:* Common. The lesion is covered with skin and fascia. Usually asymptomatic but may be mild gait or bladder problems.
  - *Cystica:* Involves herniation of the meninges (meningocoele). Uncommon but treatable, usually with minor residual defect.
  - *Whole cord herniation* (myelomeningocoele) is more common and often results in neurological deficit. It is associated with hydrocephalus, learning and psychological problems.

Primary care management
- Support the child and family. Ensure receipt of all available benefits.
- Liaise with the primary healthcare team and community and specialist services to ensure prompt provision of equipment and services.
- Tell carers about local facilities, voluntary and self-help organizations.
- Make referrals for new problems promptly.
- Liaise with specialist services to provide ongoing care.
- If the child's mother is planning another pregnancy, advise her to take 5mg folic acid od whilst planning pregnancy and until 13wk. gestation.

Genetic problems
Cleido-cranial dysostosis: Autosomal dominant inheritance. Part/all of the clavicle is missing and ossification of the skull is delayed – sutures remain open. Associated with short stature. No treatment is needed.

Osteogenesis imperfecta: Autosomal dominant inheritance (rarely recessive). Several types but all have an underlying problem with collagen metabolism, resulting in fragile bones which break easily. Other features include lax joints, thin skin, blue sclerae, hypoplastic teeth and deafness. Presentation varies according to severity. May be obvious at birth or present early with fractures. Less severe cases present later and may be mistaken for non-accidental injury. Mild cases may not present until adolescence with thin bones on x-ray. Treatment is supportive.

Osteopetrosis (marble bone disease): Autosomal dominant or recessive inheritance. Dominant form presents in childhood with fractures, osteomyelitis ± facial paralysis. Recessive form is more severe, causing bone marrow failure and death. Bone marrow transplantation has been tried but is of limited success.

Advice for patients: Information and support for parents and children

- Hypermobility Syndrome Association (HMSA):
  ⌨ www.hypermobility.org
- Association for Spina Bifida and Hydrocephalus (ASBAH):
  ☎ 01733 555 988 ⌨ www.asbah.org.uk
- Brittle Bone Society: ☎ 08000 282 459
  ⌨ www.brittlebone.org
- Osteopetrosis Support Trust: ⌨ www.ost.org.uk

GP Notes: Folate supplementation

↓ risk of neural tube defect by 72%.
- *If no previous neural tube defects:* 0.4mg od when pregnancy is being planned and for 13wk. after conception.
- *If 1 parent affected, on anti-epileptic medication or previous child affected:* 5mg od from the time the pregnancy is being planned until 13wk. after conception.

Supplements can be prescribed or are available OTC from chemists and supermarkets.

Musculoskeletal problems in childhood

Septic arthritis: Most common in children <5y. old. Tends to affect the hip or knee. The child is usually systemically unwell and holds the affected joint completely still. The joint may be swollen, hot and tender. This is an emergency – if suspected admit. Treatment is with IV antibiotics and surgical washout of the joint.

Nocturnal musculoskeletal pains (growing pains): Episodic, muscular pains – usually in the legs – lasting ~30 min. and waking the child from sleep. Rubbing the limb → rapid relief. There is no pain or disability in the morning. Diagnosis can be made on history if there are no associated symptoms and examination is normal. If in doubt, check ESR, which should be normal. In most cases reassurance ± analgesia are all that is needed. In resistant cases, physiotherapy may help.

Idiopathic musculoskeletal pain: Pain for which no cause can be found. Can become chronic. Take a history and examine carefully to exclude other causes. Investigate further only if history or examination suggest a pathological cause. Treatment is with analgesia and reassurance. Advise to return for reassessment ± orthopaedic referral if pain worsens, continues >6wk., changes in nature or other symptoms develop.

Sports injuries: 📖 p.64

Scoliosis: Lateral curvature of the spine. 2 types:
- *Structural (true) scoliosis:* Fixed deformity. Scoliosis is associated with rotation of the vertebrae ± ribs and wedging of the vertebrae.
- *Non-structural (mobile) scoliosis:* Curvature is 2° to another condition outside the spine and disappears when that is corrected – e.g. leg length disparity (disappears on sitting). No rotation of the vertebrae.

Causes of true scoliosis
- *Idiopathic:* 📖 p.32
- *Congenital:* Vertebral malformations produce severe scoliosis which is rapidly progressive. *Major causes:* Hemivertebra; Klippel-Feil syndrome; congenital vertebral bar due to failure of segmentation
- *Neuromuscular imbalance:* e.g. polio, cerebral palsy, muscular dystrophy, neurofibromatosis, syringomyelia
- *Trauma:* → in damage to the vertebral growth plate and uneven growth
- *Neoplasm:*
  - *1°:* Osteoid osteoma and osteoblastoma cause a painful scoliosis
  - *2°:* Lytic metastases
  - *Treatment* of tumours e.g. radiotherapy can → scoliosis
- *Metabolic:* Osteoporosis and crush fracture
- *Infection:* TB of the spine (Pott's disease)

Presentation: Usually found incidentally or on screening (📖 p.20).

Management: Refer children with structural scoliosis to orthopaedics.

Complications: Deformity; pain; limitation of activities; respiratory restriction

Referral guidelines for cancer in children and young people[N]:

Consider referral:
- When a child or young person presents with persistent back pain (an examination is needed and a FBC and blood film).
- When there is persistent parental anxiety, even when a benign cause is considered most likely.

Refer urgently: when a child/young person presents several times (≥3x) with the same problem, but with no clear diagnosis.

Bone sarcomas (osteosarcoma and Ewing's sarcoma): Refer children or young people with:
- rest pain, back pain and unexplained limp (a discussion with a paediatrician or X-ray should be considered before or as well as referral)
- persistent localized bone pain and/or swelling, and X-ray showing signs of cancer. In this case refer urgently.

Soft tissue sarcoma: Refer urgently a child or young person presenting with an unexplained mass at almost any site that has ≥1 of the following features:

The mass is:
- deep to the fascia
- non-tender
- progressively enlarging
- associated with a regional lymph node that is enlarging
- >2cm in diameter in size.

31

GP Notes: How can I detect scoliosis?

Look for:
- Difference in shoulder height
- Spinal curvature
- Difference in space between trunk and upper limbs

🔵 Structural scoliosis is often made more obvious by asking the child to bend forwards. Scoliosis which disappears on bending is postural and of no clinical significance.

⚠ If scoliosis is painful in a child or young person – especially at night – consider spinal tumour and refer for urgent orthopaedic assessment.

Advice for patients: Information and support

- Scoliosis Association (UK): ☎ 020 8964 1166
  🖥 www.sauk.org.uk
- Arthritis Research Campaign (ARC): ☎ 0870 8505000
  🖥 www.arc.org.uk

Further information

NICE: Referral guidelines for suspected cancer-quick reference guide (2005) 🖥 www.nice.org.uk

Idiopathic scoliosis: >10° of lateral curvature of the spine – thoracic curves tend to be more severe than lumbar. *Incidence:* 1–3%.

Infantile idiopathic scoliosis: ♂:♀≈6:4. 90% are left sided convex scolioses. Associated with ipsilateral plagiocephaly (flattening of the skull). May resolve spontaneously (more likely if ♂, onset at <1y. of age and/or the rib–vertebral angle is <20°) or progress as the child grows. Progressive scoliosis is treated with braces and surgery. As a general rule, the younger the child and the higher the curve, the worse the prognosis.

Late-onset idiopathic scoliosis: Affects children aged 10–15y. ♀:♂≈9:1. The scoliosis is usually right-sided convex. The condition always gets worse without treatment as the child grows. Treatment is with observation (if the scoliosis is mild and the child has nearly completed growth), braces and/or surgery.

Pulled elbow: Common in children <5y. Traction injury to elbow causes subluxation of radial head. Often occurs when the child is pulled up suddenly by the hand. Child will not use the arm. No clinical signs. ♂>♀. Left arm > right. X-rays are unhelpful.

Management: Apply anterior pressure with the thumb on the radial head whilst supinating and extending the forearm. Immediate recovery is seen after reduction.

Hip problems

Transient synovitis of the hip (irritable hip): The most common reason for limping in childhood. *Peak age:* 2–10y. ♂>>♀. The child is usually well but complains of pain in the hip or knee and may refuse to weight bear. Often occurs after a viral infection. Cause is unknown. Exclude septic arthritis – refer to orthopaedics. Usually resolves in 7–10d. without treatment.

Perthes' disease: Pain in the hip or knee, limp and limited hip movement developing over ~1mo. Due to avascular necrosis of the femoral head. Bilateral in 10%. *Peak age:* 4–7y. (range 3–11y.). ♂:♀≈4:1.

Management: If suspected refer for x-ray and to orthopaedics. Treatment is with rest, x-ray surveillance, bracing and/or surgery depending on severity.

Prognosis: Usually heals over 2–3y. Joint damage may lead to early arthritis. Young patients do best. Risk factors for poor outcome include:
- ♀
- Onset >8y.
- Involvement of the whole femoral head
- Pronounced metaphyseal rarefaction
- Lateral displacement of the femoral head.

GP Notes: The limping child

- If a child is limping, take it seriously and look for a problem.
- Children find it difficult to localize pain and pain can be referred from the hip to the knee, so examine the whole limb carefully.
- Other causes of referred pain include: spinal pathology, psoas spasm from GI pathology (e.g. appendicitis).
- Limping without pain is uncommon and may be due to undiagnosed congenital hip dislocation – 📖 p.26

Advice for patients: Information and support

- Scoliosis Association (UK): ☎ 020 8964 1166
  🖥 www.sauk.org.uk
- Steps Support for patients with lower limb conditions and their families: ☎ 0871 717 0044 🖥 www.steps-charity.org.uk
- Arthritis Research Campaign (ARC): ☎ 0870 850 5000
  🖥 www.arc.org.uk

Slipped upper femoral epiphysis: The upper femoral epiphysis slips with respect to the femur, usually in a postero-inferior direction. Bilateral in 20%. *Incidence:* 1:100,000. *Peak age:* 10–15y. ♂:♀≈3:1. Typically affects obese, underdeveloped children or tall, thin boys.

Presentation:
- Pain at rest in the groin, hip, thigh or referred to the knee – may be mild.
- Limp and/or pain on movement.
- ↓ hip movements – particularly abduction and medial rotation. The affected leg may be externally rotated and shortened.

Management: Confirm diagnosis on x-ray (include lateral views) – shows backwards and downwards slippage of the epiphysis. Refer to orthopaedics – surgical pinning or reconstructive surgery is needed. Monitoring of the other hip is essential.

Complications: Avascular necrosis; coxa vara; early arthritis; slipped epiphysis on the contralateral side.

Knee problems
Bow legs and knock knees

- *Genu varum (bow legs):* Outward curving of the tibia usually associated with internal tibial torsion. Except in severe cases always resolves spontaneously. Severe cases raise the possibility of rickets or other rare developmental disorders – refer for orthopaedic opinion.
- *Genu valgum (knock knees):* Common amongst 2–4y. olds. Innocent if symmetrical and independent of any other abnormality. Severe, progressive cases suggest rickets – refer for x-ray.

Osgood-Schlatter disease: 📖 p.104

Chondromalacia patellae: 📖 p.104

Foot problems
Flat feet: All babies and toddlers have flat feet. The arch develops after 2–3y. of walking. Persistent flat feet may be familial or due to joint laxity. If pain free, foot is mobile and the child develops an arch on standing on tiptoe, no action is required. Else refer to orthopaedics.

Osteochondritis: Table 2.1

Sever's disease: Apophysitis of the heel. Peak age: 8–13y. Treated with analgesia, raising the heel of the shoe a little, calf-stretching and avoiding strenuous activities for a few weeks.

In-toe and out-toe gait
- *In-toe:* Originates in the femur (persistent anteversion of the femoral neck), tibia (tibial torsion) or foot (metatarsus varus). Does not cause pain or affect mobility. Usually resolves by age 5–6y.
- *Out-toe:* Common <2y. May be unilateral. Corrects spontaneously.

Table 2.1 Osteochondritis of the foot in children and young adults

	Bone(s) involved	Features	Treatment
Kohler's disease	Navicular bone	Peak age: 3–5y. Presents with pain and tenderness over the dorsum of the mid-foot. X-ray – small navicular bone of ↑ density.	Pain usually resolves with simple analgesia and rest.
Freiberg's disease	2nd and 3rd metatarsal heads	Most common in teenagers and young adults. ♀>♂. Presents with pain in the foot on walking. The head of the metatarsal is palpable and tender. X-ray shows a wide, flat metatarsal.	Treatment is usually conservative with cushioning of shoes and simple analgesia. If severe, refer to orthopaedics. Excision of the metatarsal head may relieve pain.

Advice for patients: Information and support

- Steps Support for patients with lower limb conditions and their families ☎ 0871 717 0044 🖥 www.steps-charity.org.uk
- Arthritis Research Campaign (ARC): ☎ 0870 850 5000 🖥 www.arc.org.uk

Arthritis in children

Joint and limb pains are common in children. Arthritis is rare.

Presentation of arthritis in children

Older children: Usually present with well-localized joint pains ± hot, tender, swollen joints.

Babies and young children: May present with immobility of a joint or a limp, but the diagnosis can be extremely difficult.

Differential diagnosis of joint pains in children

- Juvenile chronic arthritis (JCA)
- Infections e.g. TB, rubella
- Rheumatic fever
- Henoch Schönlein purpura
- Traumatic arthritis
- Hypermobility syndrome
- Leukaemia
- Sickle cell disease
- SLE & connective tissue disorders
- Transient synovitis of the hip (irritable hip)
- Septic arthritis
- Perthes disease
- Slipped femoral epiphysis

Septic arthritis: 📖 p.30

Types of childhood arthritis: Table 2.2

Management of children with arthritis

- If suspected, refer urgently to paediatrics for confirmation of diagnosis.
- Once confirmed, ensure the child is referred to a specialist paediatric rheumatology unit to avoid long-term disability. These units have multidisciplinary facilities for rehabilitation, education and surgical intervention (if necessary) and support both the family and the child.
- NSAIDs and paracetamol help pain and stiffness, but corticosteroids and immunosuppressants (e.g. methotrexate) are often required for systemic disease.
- Ensure families apply for any benefits that might be available to them.
- Tell families about self-help and support groups.
- Support families in any applications made to adapt the home or school environment for the child's condition.

Patient tip: Information and support

Arthritis Research Campaign (ARC): ☎ 0870 850 5000
🖳 www.arc.org.uk

Table 2.2 Childhood arthritis

Type of arthritis	Features
Oligoarthritis or pauciarticular-onset arthritis	
Persistent:	Most common form of JCA (50–60%) but still rare. Peak age: 3y. ♀>>♂. Affects ≤4 joints, especially wrists, knees and ankles. Often asymmetrical. Associated with uveitis (often with +ve anti-nuclear antibody) which requires regular screening by slit-lamp examination – rarely causes blindness. Generally prognosis is good, with remission in 4–5 y.
Extended:	Chronic arthritis with an oligoarticular onset of the disease, which progresses to involve >4 joints. Joints tend to be stiff rather than hot and swollen.
Still's disease	10% of JCA. Affects boys and girls equally up to 5y., then girls are more commonly affected. *Presentation:* • Fever – high, swinging, early-evening temperature • Rash – pink maculopapular rash • Musculoskeletal pain – arthralgia, arthritis, myalgia • Generalized lymphadenopathy • Hepatosplenomegaly • Pericarditis ± pleurisy (uncommon) *Investigations:* Blood – ↑ ESR/CRP; FBC – ↑ neutrophils, ↑ platelets. Autoantibodies are –ve. ⚠ *Differential diagnosis:* Malignancy – particularly leukaemia or neuroblastoma); infection.
Polyarticular onset JCA	Develops with or without a preceding systemic illness at any age >1y. Usually occurs in teenagers, producing widespread joint destruction. There is symmetrical arthritis of hands, wrists, PIP joints ± DIP joints. Rheumatoid factor is usually –ve (+ve in 3% – often teen-age girls).
Juvenile spondylo-arthropathy	Affects teenage and younger boys, producing an asymmetrical arthritis of lower-limb joints. Associated with HLA-B27 and acute anterior uveitis. Represents the childhood equivalent of adult ankylosing spondylitis. ~60% of childhood sufferers develop ankylosing spondylitis later in life.
Psoriatic arthritis	Polyarthritis affecting large and small joints including fingers and toes. The arthritis can be very erosive. Psoriasis may be present in the child or a first-degree relative. 📖 p. 140

Child abuse and neglect

Defined as depriving children of their human rights. These are:
- *Being healthy:* enjoying good physical and mental health and living a healthy lifestyle
- *Staying safe:* being protected from harm and neglect
- *Enjoying and achieving:* developing broad skills for adulthood
- *Making a positive contribution:* to the community and society
- *Economic well-being:* overcoming disadvantages to achieve their full potential

Statistics: ~3/100 children are abused each year in the UK; there were 4109 reported offences of cruelty or neglect of children in England and Wales in 2002/3 and every year ~30,000 children's names are added to the child protection register in England alone.

Presentation: *Always* have a high index of suspicion. *Suspect abuse if:*
- The child discloses it
- The story is inconsistent with injuries found
- There is late presentation after an injury or lack of concern about the injury by the parent(s)
- Presentation to an unknown doctor
- Accompanying adult is not the parent or guardian
- Sibling has been a victim of abuse
- Reluctance to allow the child to be examined
- Characteristic injuries – look for marks consistent with cigarette burns; scalds (especially if symmetrical or doughnut shaped on buttocks); finger mark or bite mark bruises; perineal bruising or anogenital injury; linear marks consistent with whipping; buckle or belt marks
- Multiple injuries or old injuries co-existent with new
- Unlikely sites for injuries e.g. mouth, ears, genitalia, eyes
- Behaviour of the child is suggestive e.g. withdrawn, 'frozen watchfulness', sexually precocious behaviour, abnormal interaction between child and parents, unwilling to speak about the injury etc.
- Vaginal discharge, sexually transmitted disease or recurrent UTI in any child <14y.
- Failure to thrive, developmental delay and/or behavioural problems: neglect and/or emotional abuse are included in the differential diagnosis of failure to thrive and developmental delay. Any type of abuse may result in behavioural problems

Risk factors for child abuse

Parent/carer factors
- Mental illness
- Substance/alcohol abuse
- Being abused themselves as children or adults
- Ongoing physical illness
- Learning disabilities
- Unemployment/ impoverished living conditions

Child factors
- History of sibling abuse
- Learning, behaviour or physical problems
- Unplanned pregnancy/premature birth
- Poor attachment to parents/carers
- Environment high in criticism
- 'Looked after' children

GMS contract

| Management Indicator 1 | Individual healthcare professionals have access to information on local procedures relating to child protection | 1 point |
| Education Indicator 7 | The practice has undertaken a minimum of 12 significant event reviews in the past 3 years which could include child protection cases | Total of 4 points for 12 reviews |

Table 2.3 Classification of child abuse

PHYSICAL
Hitting, shaking, throwing, burning, suffocating, poisoning, including factitious or induced illness

EMOTIONAL
The child is made to feel worthless, afraid, unloved or inadequate (e.g. if developmentally inappropriate expectations are imposed)

NEGLECT
Failure to meet the child's basic needs, allowing the child to be exposed to danger

SEXUAL
Forcing/enticing a child to take part in sexual activities – may involve physical contact, or production of pornographic material

ⓘ In practice there is often overlap and >1 type of abuse may co-occur.

GP Notes: How to deal with child protection with confidence

- Make sure you are familiar with the practice and local child protection procedures.
- Make sure you attend child protection training regularly.
- Share your concerns with colleagues and try to use shared documentation and computer templates as much as possible.

Immediate action

⚠ Welfare of the child is *paramount*. Not to report abuse is to collude with the abuser.

- Wherever possible, arrange for another health professional to be present during the consultation.
- Take a history from any accompanying adult. If possible, also take a history from the child alone too. Do not contaminate evidence by asking leading questions.
- Fully examine the child. Ask for an explanation for any injuries noted.
- Keep thorough notes, recording dates and times, history given, injuries noted and any explanation of those injuries.

Further action: Depends on nature of the suspected abuse, suspected abuser (e.g. if someone outside the home is suspected, the child is safe to return home), nature of the injuries and response of the parents. Be familiar with and follow local guidelines and practice policy. *Options are:*

- Hospital admission – protects the child and allows full assessment.
- Liaison with social services child protection team (on-call 24h./d.).
- If admission is refused, contact social services to arrange a Place of Safety Order, or the police to take the child into police protection.
- Contact social services if your observations and discussions lead you to feel that this is a child protection issue and follow the referral up in 48h. with a written referral. You should receive confirmation of your referral within 1 but certainly within 3 working days.
- You can also refer directly to the police, particularly if you feel emergency action may be required to protect the child.

Difficult issues for health professionals in child protection

- Confidentiality of medical information
- Sharing information with parents and carers
- Fear of damaging future relationships with the family
- Fear of causing family disruption
- Fear of dealing with other agencies e.g. police and social services
- Fear of being mistaken in one's suspicions
- Fear of missing abuse
- Fear of attending court
- Fear of negative peer review

Further information

DoH: 🖥 www.dh.gov.uk
- *Working together to safeguard children* (1998)
- *What to do if you're worried a child is being abused* (2003)
RCGP: Carter & Bannon. *The role of primary care in the protection of children from abuse and neglect* (2003) 🖥 www.rcgp.org.uk
Department for Education and Skills: *Every child matters* (2004)
🖥 www.everychildmatters.gov.uk

Figure 2.2 The 4-step approach to managing child abuse

Step 1	Step 2	Step 3	Step 4
			Intervention
		Enquiry and assessment of risk	Consists of supportive and rehabilitation measures in order to enable child development.
	Reporting		
Recognition			
Health professionals either identify or suspect a situation where a child may be at risk of abuse or neglect.	Suspicions are reported or discussed with social services, police and/or child protection agencies. Concerns regarding a family become 'public' – this is often the threshold at which those in primary care hesitate and step back from the brink.	Concerns and allegations are explored, information is gathered and risk to children determined. A multi-agency approach is usually employed.	

GP Notes: Determining abuse

⚠ This guidance appears simple – and *is* when abuse is overt – but often it is *difficult* to decide if a child is being abused. If you have worries but cannot justify them sufficiently to invoke child protection procedures:
- Check via social services whether the child is on the 'at risk' register
- Check notes of siblings and other family members to see if there has been any suggestion of abuse in the family before
- Discuss your worries with the health visitor and/or other involved members of the primary health care team.

If any of these sources ↑ your suspicion, you may be justified in investigating further or invoking child protection measures at that point.

If you are still unsure what to do, record your worries and the reasons for them in the child's notes and alert all other involved members of the practice team. Review whenever that child is seen again in the practice.

Chapter 3

Injuries presenting to general practice

Road traffic accidents (RTAs)

Doctors are not legally obliged to attend an accident they happen to pass – but most feel morally obliged to do so.

Immediate action
- Assess the scene.
- Ensure police and ambulance have been called.
- Take steps to ensure your own safety and that of others: park your vehicle defensively; turn on hazard lights; use warning triangles.
- Ensure all vehicle ignitions are turned off.
- Triage casualties into priority groups: decide who to attend first.
- Forbid smoking.

Immediate treatment
- Check the need for basic resuscitation:
  - Airway patent?
  - Breathing adequate?
  - Circulation intact?
- Resuscitate as necessary (Figures 3.1 and 3.2).
- Control any haemorrhage with elevation and pressure.
- DO NOT attempt to move anyone who potentially could have a back or neck injury until skilled personnel and equipment are available.
- Do not give anything by mouth.
- Use coats and rugs to keep victims warm.
- If available give analgesia (e.g. opiates – but not if significant head injury or risk of intraperitoneal injury; entonox – from ambulance).
- If shocked set up IV fluids.
- Take directions from the paramedics – they are almost certainly more experienced than you in these situations.

Medico-legal issues
- Ensure your medico-legal insurance covers emergency treatments.
- Keep full records of events, action taken, drugs administered, origin of drugs, batch numbers and expiry dates.
- A GP can charge a fee to the victims for any assistance given.

GMS contract		
Education Indicator 1	There is a record of all practice-employed staff having attended training/updating in basic life support skills in the preceding 18mo.	4 points
Education Indicator 5	There is a record of all practice-employed staff having attended training/updating in basic life support skills in the preceding 36mo.	3 points

Figures 3.1 and 3.2 are reproduced from the Resuscitation guidelines (2005) with permission of the Resuscitation Council (UK) 🖫 www.resus.org.uk

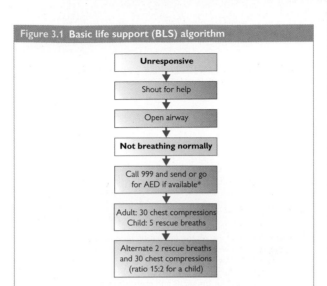

Figure 3.1 Basic life support (BLS) algorithm

Unresponsive

↓

Shout for help

↓

Open airway

↓

Not breathing normally

↓

Call 999 and send or go
for AED if available*

↓

Adult: 30 chest compressions
Child: 5 rescue breaths

↓

Alternate 2 rescue breaths
and 30 chest compressions
(ratio 15:2 for a child)

* For children, perform CPR for 1 minute before going for help

Reproduced with permission of the Resuscitation Council (UK).

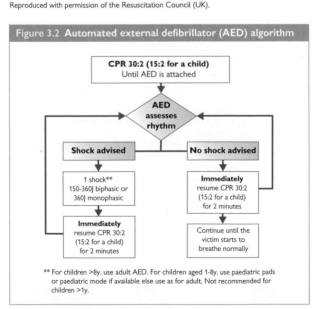

Figure 3.2 Automated external defibrillator (AED) algorithm

CPR 30:2 (15:2 for a child)
Until AED is attached

↓

**AED
assesses
rhythm**

Shock advised | **No shock advised**

1 shock**
150-360J biphasic or
360J monophasic

Immediately
resume CPR 30:2
(15:2 for a child)
for 2 minutes

Immediately
resume CPR 30:2
(15:2 for a child)
for 2 minutes

Continue until the
victim starts to
breathe normally

** For children >8y. use adult AED. For children aged 1-8y. use paediatric pads
or paediatric mode if available else use as for adult. Not recommended for
children >1y.

Reproduced with permission of the Resuscitation Council (UK).

Common injuries and accidents

Wounds: Most patients with significant lacerations present directly to A&E. If a patient presents to general practice, perform immediate care (elevate bleeding limb and apply pressure to arrest bleeding). Advise nil by mouth and transfer to A&E.

Minor lacerations

- Ensure no foreign body is in the wound – if in doubt refer for x-ray/surgical exploration (especially important if injury was with glass).
- Wash wound and clean away debris and any necrotic material.
- Check there is no damage to underlying nerves, tendons, bone or blood supply before dressing or closing a wound.
- Aim to oppose the skin edges without tension to allow healing.
- Do not attempt to close a wound if you are not confident that you can achieve an adequate result.
- Always refer cuts through the lip margin to A&E; consider referral to A&E for any facial wounds and wounds in children.
- Check tetanus status (Figure 3.3).
- In assault cases take particular care to document all injuries carefully e.g. with photographs, drawings and measurements of wounds.
- Consider non-accidental injury in children – 📖 p.38.

Closing the wound: *Options:*

Skin closure strips (Steristrips): use for small cuts in non-hairy skin not under tension. Can also be used in addition to sutures for larger wounds.

Skin 'glue' (e.g. Histoacryl): quick (takes 30sec. to set) and can be used on hairy skin such as the scalp.

Suturing: Undertake training before attempting suturing.
- Infiltrate wound edges with 1% lidocaine (max. 2mg/kg).
- Addition of adrenaline (epinephrine) can help haemostasis but must not be used on digits or extremities as necrosis can occur.
- Take care to oppose edges accurately – start interrupted sutures in the middle of the wound.
- Use appropriate suture (e.g. adult face 5-0 monofilament nylon – remove after 5d.; limbs or trunk 3–0 nylon – remove after 1–2wk.).

Pretibial lacerations: The shin has poor blood supply, especially in the elderly. Flap wounds are common, may heal poorly ± break down to form ulcers. *Management:* Wash the wound. Carefully realign the flap, secure with steristrips without tension and bandage. Advise elevation of the leg. Review regularly to check healing.

Subungual haematoma: 📖 p.94

Air gun pellets: Common. Refer for x-ray. Can be difficult to remove and may be left in place if not in a harmful position. If in a joint refer for removal.

Fish hooks: Infiltrate with lidocaine. Push the hook forwards through the skin until the barb is exposed. Cut the barb off and then ease the hook back through the skin the same way it entered.

Figure 3.3 Who should have tetanus vaccination?

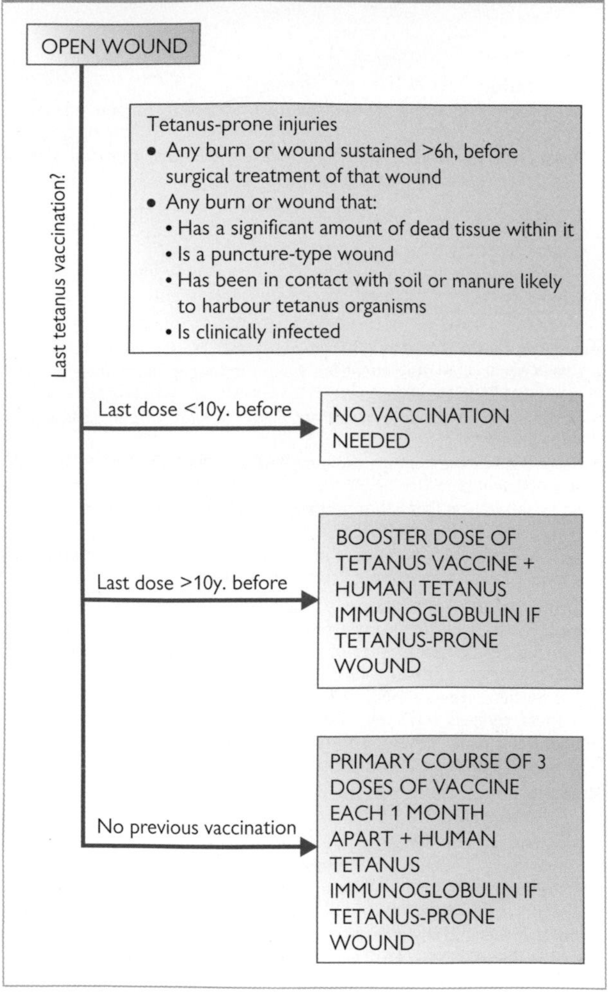

OPEN WOUND

Last tetanus vaccination?

Tetanus-prone injuries
- Any burn or wound sustained >6h, before surgical treatment of that wound
- Any burn or wound that:
  - Has a significant amount of dead tissue within it
  - Is a puncture-type wound
  - Has been in contact with soil or manure likely to harbour tetanus organisms
  - Is clinically infected

Last dose <10y. before → NO VACCINATION NEEDED

Last dose >10y. before → BOOSTER DOSE OF TETANUS VACCINE + HUMAN TETANUS IMMUNOGLOBULIN IF TETANUS-PRONE WOUND

No previous vaccination → PRIMARY COURSE OF 3 DOSES OF VACCINE EACH 1 MONTH APART + HUMAN TETANUS IMMUNOGLOBULIN IF TETANUS-PRONE WOUND

Fractures

Presentation
- *Symptoms:* Pain at the affected site made worse by movement; loss of function
- *Signs:* Swelling; bruising; deformity; local tenderness; impaired function; crepitus; abnormal mobility

> **Action:**
> - Immobilize the affected part and give analgesia.
> - If available and the patient is shocked, start an IV infusion.
> - Refer to A&E for assessment, x-ray and treatment.

Fracture complications
- Often occur after the patient has been discharged from hospital and may present to the GP.
- Patients should not have persistent pain – beware of compartment syndrome.
- Refer back to the fracture clinic or A&E if:
  - Persistent pain
  - Limb swelling that is not settling
  - Offensive odour or discharge
  - If cast edges are abrading the skin or if the cast has deteriorated in structural strength e.g. from getting wet.

Compartment syndrome: Crush injury, fracture, prolonged immobility or tight splints, dressings or casts can result in ↑ pressure within muscle compartments ultimately leading to vascular occlusion. Hypoxia and necrosis cause further ↑ pressure.
Signs: Swelling, severe pain – ↑ on passive stretch of muscles, distal numbness, redness, mottling, blisters 🔴 pulses may be present distally.
Action: Refer as an emergency for orthopaedic assessment – a fasciotomy may be needed to relieve the pressure.

Knocked out teeth: Ask the patient to suck tooth clean, reinsert or store in milk and send to a dentist.

Coin and other foreign body ingestion: Most coins will pass through the gut without any problems. If asymptomatic, they can be left to take their course (advise checking stools to ensure passed). If symptomatic, refer for x-ray and consideration for endoscopic removal. If there is any indication of aspiration refer urgently.

Foreign bodies in the ear: Most common in children. Try to remove under direct vision with forceps but avoid pushing objects deeper into the canal and causing damage. Don't poke around with forceps in an unco-operative child. Removal under GA may be needed. Insects can be drowned in oil and syringed out.

Foreign bodies in the nose: Common in young children. Refer all children with unilateral offensive discharge for exploration under GA. Do not try to remove a foreign body yourself unless the object is very superficial and the child co-operative. You might push the object further in and cause trauma.

GP Notes: Removing a tight ring from a swollen finger

- Wind cotton tape around the finger advancing towards the ring.
- Then thread tape through the ring and pull on this end to unwind the tape (levers ring over PIP joint).
- If unsuccessful, use a ring cutter.

Animal bites: ~200,000 people are bitten by dogs each year in the UK. Animal bites are contaminated and wound infection is common. Clean carefully with soap and water. Check tetanus status. Do not suture unless cosmetically essential and there is minimal tissue damage – refer if in doubt. Give prophylaxis against infection (e.g. with co-amoxiclav or erythromycin).

Human bites: especially prone to infection. Also consider risk of hepatitis B and HIV. If HIV prophylaxis is indicated, it needs to be started immediately–refer urgently to A&E for local policy implementation.

Snake bites: The adder is the only poisonous snake in the UK. Bites are only rarely lethal. Attempt to identify the snake species and refer the patient urgently to hospital. Do not apply a tourniquet or try cutting or sucking the wound.

Insect stings: Response depends on the insect involved and the individual's response to the stings. Ranges from blisters through papules to urticarial wheals – 2° infection is common.

Management

Anaphylaxis: Follow algorithm in Figure 3.4 and admit to hospital as a blue-light emergency.

Immediately after the sting: Remove any sting present in the wound; often no further treatment is needed.

- *If severe local reaction occurs:* Apply an ice pack; give oral antihistamine (e.g. chlorphenamine 4mg stat); continue antihistamine 4–6 hourly as needed.
- *If 2° bacterial infection occurs:* Treat with oral or topical antibiotics.

Remove sources of insects e.g. remove fleas from carpets with household flea spray (multiple bites on ankles and lower legs).

Removal of ticks: Place a large blob of petroleum jelly (Vaseline™) over the tick. It suffocates over a few hours and can be removed easily with a pair of tweezers.

Weaver fish sting: Common on sandy beaches. The fish lurks under the sand so usually trodden on – presents with severe pain in the foot. Immerse the affected area in uncomfortably hot (but not scalding) water. Give analgesia. Pain resolves after 2–3d.

Jelly fish sting
- Remove the patient from the sea as soon as possible.
- Scrape or wash adherent tentacles off.
- Alcoholic solutions including suntan lotions should not be applied because they may cause further discharge of stinging hairs.
- Ice packs ↓ pain and a slurry of baking soda (sodium bicarbonate), but not vinegar, may be useful for treating stings from UK species.

GMS contract		
Medicines Indicator 2	The practice possesses the equipment and indate emergency drugs to treat anaphylaxis	2 points

Figure 3.4 Emergency treatment of anaphylaxis

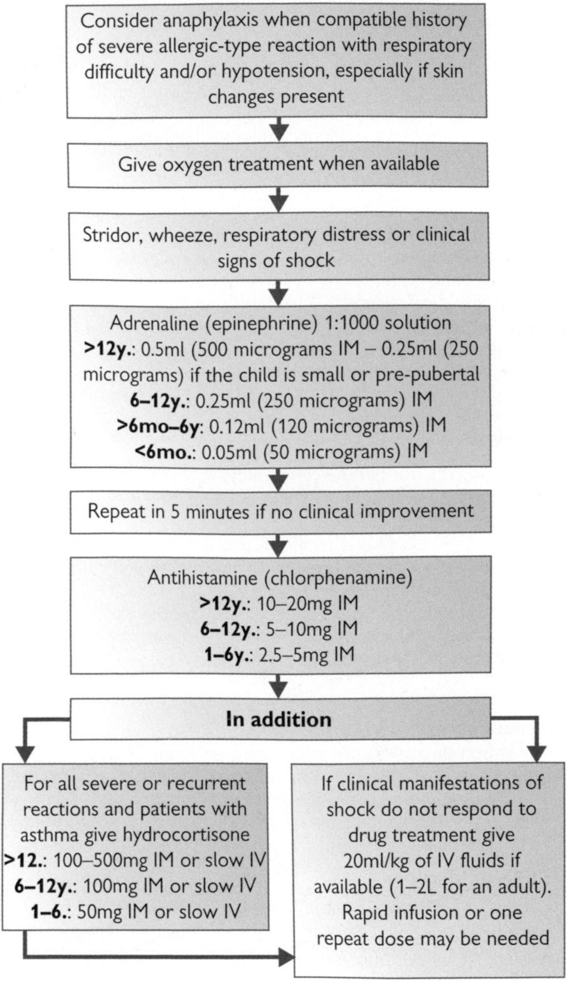

Consider anaphylaxis when compatible history of severe allergic-type reaction with respiratory difficulty and/or hypotension, especially if skin changes present

↓

Give oxygen treatment when available

↓

Stridor, wheeze, respiratory distress or clinical signs of shock

↓

Adrenaline (epinephrine) 1:1000 solution
>12y.: 0.5ml (500 micrograms IM – 0.25ml (250 micrograms) if the child is small or pre-pubertal
6–12y.: 0.25ml (250 micrograms) IM
>6mo–6y: 0.12ml (120 micrograms) IM
<6mo.: 0.05ml (50 micrograms) IM

↓

Repeat in 5 minutes if no clinical improvement

↓

Antihistamine (chlorphenamine)
>12y.: 10–20mg IM
6–12y.: 5–10mg IM
1–6y.: 2.5–5mg IM

↓

In addition

For all severe or recurrent reactions and patients with asthma give hydrocortisone
>12.: 100–500mg IM or slow IV
6–12y.: 100mg IM or slow IV
1–6.: 50mg IM or slow IV

If clinical manifestations of shock do not respond to drug treatment give 20ml/kg of IV fluids if available (1–2L for an adult). Rapid infusion or one repeat dose may be needed

51

Reproduced with permission of the Resuscitation Council UK.

Scalds and burns: *Assess:*
- Cause, size and thickness of the burn.
- Use the 'Rule of Nines' to estimate the extent of the burn (Box 3.1).
- Partial thickness burns are red, painful and blistered; full thickness burns are painless and white or grey.
- Always consider non-accidental injury in children – 📖 p.38.

⚠ Action
- Remove clothing from the affected area and place under cold running water for >10min. or until pain is relieved.
- Do not burst blisters.
- Prescribe/give analgesia.
- Refer all but the smallest (<5%) partial thickness burns for assessment in A&E.
- Refer all electrical burns for assessment in A&E.
- Refer all chemical burns for assessment in A&E unless burn area is minimal and pain free.
- Consider referral to A&E for smoke inhalation.

If managing the burn in the community:
- Check tetanus immunity and give immunization ± prophylaxis as necessary – 📖 p.47.
- Apply silver sulfadiazine cream (Flamazine) or vaseline impregnated gauze and non-adherent dressings and review for healing and infection every 1–2d.
- Cover burns on hands in Flamazine and place in a plastic bag. Elevate the hand in a sling and encourage finger movement.
- Refer if burns are not healed in 10–12 d.

Prevention of scalds and burns
- Prevention through public education is important.
- Children often sustain burns by pulling on the flex of boiling kettles or irons, pulling on saucepan handles or climbing onto hot cookers.
- Refer any children who have sustained accidental burns to the health visitor for follow-up.

Smoke inhalation
- Refer all patients who have potentially inhaled smoke for assessment – a seemingly well patient can deteriorate later.
- Smoke can cause thermal injury, carbon monoxide poisoning and cyanide poisoning.
- Airway problems occur due to thermal and chemical damage to the airways causing oedema – suspect if singed nasal hairs, a sore throat or a hoarse voice.
- Carbon monoxide poisoning may result in the classic cherry-red mucosa – but this may be absent.
- Cyanide poisoning is commonly due to smouldering plastics and causes dizziness, headaches and seizures.

Box 3.1 Rule of Nines

Ignore areas of erythema only.

Palm	1%
Arm (all over)	9%
Leg (all over)	18% (14% children)
Front	18%
Back	18%
Head (all over)	9% (14% children)
Genitals	1%

⚠ The Rule of Nines is inaccurate for children <10y. For children and for small burns, an alternative method is to estimate the extent of the burn by comparison with the area of the patient's hand. The area of the fingers and palm ≈ 1% total body surface area burn.

GP Notes: Burns in special situations

Chemical burns
- Usually caused by strong acids or alkalis.
- Wear gloves to remove contaminated clothing.
- Irrigate with cold running water for ≥20 min.
- Do not attempt to neutralise the chemical – this can exacerbate injury by producing heat.
- Refer all burns to A&E unless the burn area is minimal and pain free.

Electric shock
- Causes thermal tissue injury and direct injury due to the electric current passing through the tissue.
- Skin burns may be seen at the entry and exit site of the current.
- Muscle damage can be severe with minimal skin injury.
- Cardiac damage may occur and rhabdomyolysis can lead to renal failure.
- Refer all patients for specialist management.

Head injury

Severe head injury
- Perform basic life support (📖 p.45).
- Protect the cervical spine (see below and 📖 p.70).
- Transfer to A&E by ambulance.

Less severe head injuries

History: If possible take the history from a witness as well as the patient. Ask about circumstances of injury, loss of consciousness (LOC), seizures, current symptoms and behaviour.

Examination: Check scalp, head for injury, neurological examination (including fundi), other injuries – accompanying neck injuries are common.

⚠ *Refer to A&E if*[N]
- Glasgow Coma Scale <15 at any time since injury (Table 3.1)
- Loss of consciousness
- Focal neurological deficit since injury – problems speaking, understanding, reading, writing, ↓ sensation, loss of balance, weakness, visual changes, abnormal reflexes, problems walking, irritability or altered behaviour especially in young children
- Any suspicion of skull fracture; penetrating head injury; blood or CSF in the nose, ear or wound; serious scalp laceration or haematoma
- Amnesia for events before or after injury
- Persistent headache
- Vomiting
- Seizure
- Any previous cranial neurosurgical interventions
- High-energy head injury (e.g. pedestrian hit by motor vehicle, fall >1m or >5 stairs)
- History of bleeding or clotting disorder or on anticoagulant therapy
- Difficulty in assessing the patient (e.g. very young, elderly, intoxicated or epileptic) or concern about diagnosis
- Suspicion of non-accidental injury
- Inadequate supervision at home

If there is a history of neck pain/neck injury, immobilize the neck and refer to A&E.

If examination is normal

- Warn the patient (+ carer) they may suffer mild headaches, tiredness, dizziness, tinnitus, poor concentration and poor memory for the next few days.
- Advise rest and paracetamol (but not codeine-based analgesics) for the headache.
- Young children can be difficult to assess – sleepiness is common and not a worrying sign as long as the child is rousable.
- Give written head injury information regarding warning signs to trigger reconsultation – drowsiness, severe headache, persistent vomiting, visual disturbance and/or unusual behaviour.

Table 3.1 The Glasgow Coma Scale

Eye opening:	Spontaneous	4
	To voice	3
	To pain	2
	None	1
Best verbal response:	Oriented	5
	Confused	4
	Inappropriate words	3
	Incomprehensive	2
	none	1
Best motor response:	Obeys command	6
	Localizes pain	5
	Withdraw	4
	Flexion	3
	Extension	2
	None	1

Total score = eye opening + best verbal + best motor response scores

GP Notes: ❶ Watch out for post-concussion syndrome

Seen following even quite minor head injury. Due to neuronal damage.

Features include all or some of:
- Headache
- Dizziness
- Poor concentration
- Fatigue
- Depression
- Memory problems

Treatment is supportive and symptoms usually resolve with time (though can take months or even years).

Further information

NICE: *Triage, assessment investigation and early management of head injury in infants, children and adults* (2003) ⊞ www.nice.org.uk

Advice for patients: Advice card for people who have sustained a head injury and/or their carers

We think that it is all right for you to leave the surgery now. We have checked your symptoms and you seem well on the road to recovery.

When you get home it is very unlikely that you will have any further problems. But if any of the following symptoms do return we suggest you get someone to take you to your nearest hospital A&E department as soon as possible:

- Unconsciousness, or lack of full consciousness (for example, problems keeping eyes open)
- Any confusion (not knowing where you are, getting things muddled up)
- Any drowsiness (feeling sleepy) that goes on longer than 1 hour when you would normally be wide awake
- Difficulty waking up
- Any problems understanding or speaking
- Any loss of balance or problems walking
- Any weakness in one or more arms or legs
- Any problems with your eyesight
- Very painful headaches that won't go away
- Any vomiting or getting sick
- Any fits (collapsing or passing out suddenly)
- Clear fluid coming out of your ear or nose
- New bleeding from one or both ears
- New deafness in one or both ears

Things you shouldn't worry about: You may experience some other symptoms over the next few days which should disappear in the next 2 weeks. These include:

- Mild headache
- Feeling sick (without vomiting)
- Dizziness
- Irritability or bad temper
- Problems concentrating
- Problems with your memory
- Tiredness
- Lack of appetite
- Problems sleeping

If you feel very concerned about any of these symptoms in the first few days, you should come back and see your GP to talk about them.

If these problems do not go away after 2 weeks, you should make an appointment to see your GP.

Long-term problems: Most people recover quickly from their accident and experience no long-term problems. However, a few people develop problems after weeks or months. If you start to feel that things are not quite right (for example, memory problems, not feeling yourself), then please contact your doctor as soon as possible so that he/she can make sure you are recovering properly.

Advice for patients: Contd.

Things that will help you get better: If you follow this advice you should get better more quickly and it may help any symptoms you have to go away.

- **DO NOT** stay at home alone for the first 48 hours after your head injury.
- **DO** make sure you stay within easy reach of a telephone and medical help.
- **DO** have plenty of rest and avoid stressful situations.
- **DO NOT** take sleeping pills, sedatives or tranquillizers unless you have checked with your doctor first that it is alright to do so.
- **DO NOT** play any contact sport (for example, rugby or football) for at least 3 weeks without talking to your doctor first.
- **DO NOT** return to your normal school, college or work activity until you feel you have completely recovered.
- **DO NOT** drive a car or motorbike, ride a bicycle, or operate machinery unless you feel you have completely recovered.

⚠ If you have any effects lasting more than a few days, seek your doctor's opinion about your ability to drive a car or motorbike before driving.

TELEPHONE NUMBER TO CALL IF YOU ARE WORRIED
020 7067 5800 (NICE)

Reproduced in modified form with permission from NICE: *Triage, assessment, investigation and early management of head injury in infants, children and adults* (2003) ▣ www.nice.org.uk

Injury to the face: Mostly due to RTAs and violent incidents.
- Document injuries – your notes may be required for legal proceedings.
- Look for other injuries e.g. airway problems, head injury, neck injury.
- Palpate the face for signs of a fracture – if present refer to maxillofacial surgeons for assessment.
- Check tetanus status.
- Post-traumatic stress disorder is common after facial injury.

> ⚠ **Neurological assessment** is required if the patient has had a head injury or loss of consciousness.
>
> Always look for associated fractures of the zygoma and maxillary bones ('step' deformity in the orbit, dental malocclusion, difficulty opening the jaw, diplopia) and refer urgently to maxillofacial surgeon if present.

Specific injuries

Fractured mandible: A blow to the jaw can cause unilateral or bilateral fractures.

Signs: Presents with pain (worse on moving jaw), bruising ± bleeding inside the mouth ± discontinuity of the teeth (displaced fracture) ± numbness of the lower lip (if the inferior dental nerve has been damaged).

Action: Refer for x-ray via A&E.

Dislocated jaw: Presents with pain and the mouth is stuck open – refer for x-ray and reduction via maxillofacial surgeons or A&E.

Fractured zygoma/malar complex: A blow on the cheek may fracture the zygomatic arch in isolation or more usually cause a 'tripod' fracture.

Signs: Bony tenderness, flattening of the malar process – best seen from above (may be masked by swelling), epistaxis, subconjunctival haemorrhage extending posteriorly and infraorbital numbness, ± jaw locked.

Action: Refer for x-ray via A&E. Advise not to blow nose.

'Blow out' fracture of orbit: Uncommon fracture due to blunt trauma to the eye (e.g. squash ball injury).

Signs: Enophthalmos (may be masked by swelling), infraorbital nerve loss and inability to look upwards due to trapping of inferior rectus muscle.

Action: Refer for x-ray and assessment of eye trauma via A&E.

Middle third facial fractures (Le Fort): Usually bilateral.

Signs: Epistaxis, CSF rhinorrhea, crepitus on palpation, swelling, open bite and risk of airway compromise

Action: Refer for x-ray via A&E.

Nasal fracture: Undisplaced nasal fractures can usually be allowed to heal without intervention. X-rays are unhelpful.

Action:

- Give adequate analgesia and advise that bruising may be extensive and the nose will feel blocked for 1–2wk.
- Assessment for permanent deformity can be difficult at the time of the injury due to soft tissue swelling – reassess 7–10d. after injury.
- Refer any patient with significant deformity, or if the patient is unhappy with the appearance of their nose, to the ENT department for reduction under GA. Ideally reduction should take place within 1–2wk. (and max. 3wk.) after fracture – so refer promptly.
- Deviation of the nasal septum may not be correctable at the time of manipulation and if symptomatic will need a later submucous resection.

CSF rhinorrhoea or otorrhoea: Clear fluid dripping from the nose or ear after trauma can indicate a fracture and CSF leak. Fluid tests +ve for glucose. It suggests significant trauma – refer to A&E for head injury assessment. Spontaneous healing of the CSF leak is the norm but if it persists refer to neurosurgery for assessment for dural closure.

Septal haematoma: May occur after nasal injury and causes nasal blockage. Presents as a bilateral soft bulging of the septum. Refer urgently to ENT for evacuation to prevent cartilage destruction.

Haematoma of the pinna: Usually after trauma (e.g. rugby). Must be evacuated urgently (aspirated via large-bore needle or surgically) to prevent necrosis of the cartilage and 'cauliflower' ear – refer to ENT.

Falls amongst the elderly

Falls are a major cause of disability and the leading cause of mortality due to injury in people aged >75y. The government sets out its strategy for tackling falls in the National Service Framework for Older People. The key interventions proposed include public health strategies to ↓ incidence of falls in the population and identification, assessment and prevention measures for those most at risk of falling.

Incidence: ↑ with age – 1:3 adults >65y. living in the community have fallen in the past year and ½ of those living in institutions.

Risk factors for falls: Recurrent falls ↑ with number of risk factors:

- ♀:♂ ≈ 2:1 in the over –75s
- ↑ age
- Multiple previous falls
- Disorders of gait or balance
- Visual impairment
- Cognitive impairment
- Low morale/depression
- High level of dependence
- ↓ mobility
- Lower limb weakness or arthritis
- Foot problems
- History of stroke or PD
- Use of psychotropic drugs, sedatives, diuretics or β-blockers
- Alcohol
- Environmental factors (e.g. loose rugs, poor lighting, ice on the pavement, high winds)
- Infection – pneumonia, UTI

History: Deal with the injuries first – ask about pain, loss of function, headache. Ask carers about behaviour.

Examination: Check for bruising, loss of function, confusion, BP, pulse, neurology and fundi. Consider hypothermia if on the floor any length of time.

Investigate the cause of the fall: *Consider:*

- *Physical problems:* neurological problems (e.g. stroke); visual loss; cardiac abnormalities (e.g. arrythmia, postural hypotension); muscular abnormalities (e.g. steroid-induced myopathy); skeletal problems (e.g. osteoarthritis).
- *Environmental problems:* climbing ladders to do routine maintenance; loose/holed carpets; slippery floor or bath; chair or bed too low.

Management

- Treat any acute injury. ❶ Subdural haematoma may take several days or weeks to reveal itself.
- Perform a falls assessment (📖 p.62) or refer to a specialist falls service for a falls assessment.
- Undertake measures to ↓ risk of falls/damage from falling – 📖 p.62
- Specialist referral to the care-of-the-elderly team is appropriate if:
  - The cause of recurrent falls remains unclear
  - The patient or carer is worried about the possibility of further falls *or*
  - There is doubt about whether the patient can cope in their current social circumstances.

Box 3.2 Consequences of falling

- 20% who experience a fall will incur an injury requiring acute medical attention, though <1:10 falls result in a fracture (mainly Colles' and fractured neck of femur).
- Even if uninjured, older people might not be able to get up off the floor without help. The result may be a prolonged period of lying on the floor until help arrives. Apart from the indignity and helplessness this generates, secondary problems e.g. pneumonia, pressure sores, hypothermia and dehydration may follow.
- Any fall may seriously undermine an elderly person's confidence and make them (and their relatives/carers) worry about the possibility of recurrence. As a result, they may restrict activities, becoming less fit and more dependent on others.

Advice for patients: Information and support for patients

- Disabled Living Foundation: 🖥 www.dlf.org.uk
- Royal Society for the Prevention of Accidents:
  🖥 www.rospa.co.uk

Further information

Bandolier: *Falls in the elderly* 🖥 www.jr2.ox.ac.uk/bandolier/band20/b20-5.html

Cochrane: Gillespie *et al. Interventions for preventing falls in elderly people* (2002)

British Geriatric Society Falls and Bone Health Special Interest Group: 🖥 www.falls-and-bone-health.org.uk

SIGN: *Prevention and management of hip fracture in older people* (2002) 🖥 www.sign.ac.uk

NICE: *Guidelines for the assessment and prevention of falls* (2004) 🖥 www.nice.org.uk

Feder *et al.* (2000) Guidelines for the prevention of falls in people over 65. *BMJ.* 321: 1007–11. 🖥 www.bmj.com

National Service Framework for Older People: 🖥 www.dh. gov.uk

Prevention of falls: Falls are one of the biggest risk factors for fracture. Tendency to fall ↑ with age. All elderly people should have their risk of falls assessed regularly, whether or not they have osteoporosis. If they are at high risk of falling, they should then have a formal falls assessment.

Falls assessment: If available, refer to a specialist falls service. *Record:*

- Frequency and history of circumstances around any previous falls
- Drug therapy: polypharmacy, hypnotics, sedatives, diuretics, antihypertensives may all cause falls
- Assessment of vision
- Examination of gait and balance, including abnormalities due to foot problems or arthritis, and motor disorders e.g. stroke, Parkinson's disease
- Examination of basic neurological function, including mental status (impaired cognition and depression), muscle strength, lower extremity peripheral nerves, proprioception and reflexes
- Assessment of basic cardiovascular status, including BP (exclude postural hypotension), heart rate and rhythm
- Assessment of environmental risk factors e.g. poor lighting particularly on the stairs, loose carpets or rugs, badly fitting footwear or clothing, lack of safety equipment such as grab rails, steep stairs, slippery floors, or inaccessible lights or windows.

Measures to ↓ risk of falls and damage from falling

- Modify identified hazards or risk factors.
- Assess and correct vision, if possible.
- Correct postural hypotension – alter medication; consider compression stockings – but many elderly people cannot apply stockings tight enough to be of any use themselves.
- Treat other medical conditions e.g. refer to cardiology if arrythmia.
- Review medication and discontinue/alter inappropriate medication.
- Remove environmental hazards – arrange bath at a day centre, refer to OT to identify and correct hazards in the home e.g. remove loose carpets, wheeled trolley for use indoors, commode or urine bottle for night-time use, moving the bed downstairs etc.
- Refer to OT to identify and correct hazards in the home.
- Liaise with other members of the primary health care team and social services to provide additional support if needed; refer to local council for 'carephone' or alarm system to call for help if any further falls.
- Refer to rehabilitation/physiotherapy to improve confidence after falls and for weight-bearing exercise (focusing on strength and flexibility) and balance training (↓ risk of falls).
- Use of hip protectors. ↓ fracture risk in patients at high risk but compliance is a problem.[c]

Osteoporosis and prevention of fracture: 🔖 p.120

GP Notes: Is a formal falls assessment needed?

Ask if patients fall: they may not volunteer the information spontaneously. If a patient admits to falls, or you have evidence of falls from the notes, he/she needs a formal falls assessment.

The 'get up and go test': People who can get up from a chair without using their arms, walk several paces and return with no difficulty or unsteadiness are at low risk of falling and probably don't need a formal falls assessment.

The 'walking and talking test': People who have to stop walking while talking are at higher risk of falls and require a falls assessment.

Sports injuries

Principles of managing sporting injuries
- *First aid* (**A**irway, **B**reathing, **C**irculation): Refer severe injuries to A&E.
- *R I C E*
  - **R**est Relative rest of affected part whilst continuing other activities to maintain overall fitness.
  - **I**ce *and analgesia* Use immediately after injury (wrap ice in a towel and use for maximum 10min. at a time to prevent acute cold injury).
  - **C**ompression Taping or strapping can be used to treat (↓ swelling) and also to prevent acute sprains and strains.
  - **E**levation ↓ local swelling and dependent oedema, enabling quicker recovery.
- *Confirm the diagnosis:* Clinical examination, x-ray.
- *Early treatment:* according to cause. Don't delay.
- *Liaise:* with sports physician, sports physio and coach if elite athlete.
- *Rehabilitation:* Regaining fitness, strength and flexibility, examine and correct the cause of the injury (e.g. poor technique, equipment).
- *Graded return to activity:* Discuss with coach.
- *Prevention:* Suitable preparation and training (e.g. suitable footwear, warm-up and warm-down exercises, safety equipment) can ↓ likelihood of injuries.

Muscle injuries
- *Haematoma* within or between muscles can → dramatic whole limb bruising (due to tracking of blood) and stiffness. Treat with RICE regime, encourage movement in pain-free range.
- *Strain* (e.g. hamstring injury) Refer to physiotherapy. A secondary injury is likely if the patient returns to sport too soon.

Ligament injuries (sprains)
- *Grade1* – local tenderness, normal joint movement. Give NSAIDs, support strain, encourage mobilization.
- *Grade2* – slightly abnormal joint movement. More joint protection, NSAIDs, elevate limb, encourage middle of the range movement.
- *Grade 3* – abnormal joint movement. Refer to orthopaedics.

Overuse injuries: Incidence is increasing due to increasingly intensive training regimes, even amongst amateurs and especially in young athletes.
- *Causes:* Load too great for conditions, poor technique or posture, faulty or poor quality equipment.
- *Types of injury:* Stress fractures, joint tenderness or effusion, ligament and tendon strains, muscle stiffness. Overtraining syndrome – 📖 p.156.
- *Management:* Rest, NSAIDs, physiotherapy, improved training regime.
- *Prevention:* Recognize and correct poor posture or technique, check equipment is appropriate and fits, warm up and stretching before exercise, gradually ↑ intensity and duration of training.

GP Notes: Children and sports injuries

- Exercise is good for children — it stimulates development of the musculoskeletal and cardiovascular systems.
- It should be fun and not physically or emotionally over-demanding.
- Children are more prone to sports injuries due to continuing growth (bone growth plates are prone to damage) but are more flexible so have ↓ injury rate.
- Children's temperature control is not as good as adults.
- Equipment must be checked regularly to ensure it fits.
- Encourage warm-up and stretching exercises before sport.

Refer children with suspected overuse or sports injuries, which don't recover rapidly with simple analgesia, for specialist assessment — especially injuries of growth plates to ensure correct alignment and continued growth.

Further information

British Association of Sport and Exercise Medicine:
🖳 www.basem.co.uk
BMJ Publishing: ABC of sports medicine (1999) ISBN 072 791 3662

Environmental factors

- **Heat cramps:** Painful spasm of heavily exercised muscles (calves and feet) – due to salt depletion. *Treatment:* Rest, massage of affected muscle and fluid and salt replacement (e.g. dioralyte).
- **Heat stroke/exhaustion:** Exercising in excessive heat → salt and water depletion, dehydration and metabolite accumulation. *Signs:* Headache, nausea, confusion, inco-ordination, cramps, weakness, dizziness and malaise. Eventually thermoregulatory mechanisms fail → seizures and coma. *Signs:* Flushing, sweating and dehydration. Temperature may be normal (mild cases) or ↑. *Treatment:* Rest, fluid and salt replacement (e.g. dioralyte). Admission for IV fluids and supportive measures in severe cases.
- **Hypothermia:** Ensure appropriate clothing and limit time in the cold. *Signs:* Behaviour change, inco-ordination, clouding of consciousness. *Treatment:* Remove from cold environment, wrap in blankets (including the head) and transfer to hospital. Do not use direct heat.
- **Frost bite:** Freezing of the peripheries (usually feet, hands, ears or nose). Tissues become hard, insensitive and white. *Treatment:* Gentle rewarming, Refer if significant dead tissue. Debridement is usually delayed to allow natural recovery.
- **Diving:** Decompression illness is due to rapid ascent causing nitrogen dissolved in blood to form gas bubbles. Usually <1h.–36h. after surfacing. Presentation: Deep muscle aches and joint pains, skin pain, paraesthesia, itching and burning, retrosternal pain, cough and breathlessness, neurological symptoms. Refer suspected cases urgently to A&E.

'Scrumpox' (herpes gladiatorum): Herpes simplex virus is very contagious and outbreaks among sporting teams are common e.g. spread by close contact and facial stubble grazes whilst scrumming. *Treatment:* Aciclovir (cream or tablets) and exclusion of infected players. Impetigo, erysipelas and tinea barbare can be transmitted in the same way and are also sometimes called 'scrumpox'.

Fitness to perform sporting activities: GPs are commonly asked to certify fitness to perform sports. Normally the patient will come with a medical form. If there is a form, request to see it before the medical. If there is no form and you are unsure what to check, telephone the sport's governing body or the event organizer. A fee is payable by the patient.

Many gyms and sports clubs also ask older patients and patients with pre-existing conditions or disabilities to check with their GP before they will sign them on. Assuming that a suitable regime is undertaken, most people can participate in some form of sporting activity. Consider the patient's baseline fitness, check BP and medications and recommend a gradual introduction to any new forms of exercise.

⚠ *Hypertrophic obstructive cardiomyopathy* can cause sudden death during sport. It is difficult to exclude on clinical examination – if there is a FH or systolic murmur, refer to cardiology before recommending new intense activity.

GP Notes: Drugs and sport

Fitness to perform sporting activities

⚠ Remember – signing a form may result in legal action against you should the patient NOT be fit to undertake an activity.

Where possible include a caveat e.g. 'Based on information available in the medical notes the patient appears to be fit to ..., although it is impossible to guarantee this.'

If unsure, consult your local LMC or medical defence organization for advice.

Drugs and sport: Most sport regulating bodies have strict codes regarding drug use by participating sportsmen. Although broadly similar, regulations may differ in detail.

Prohibited classes of drugs
- *Stimulants:* e.g. amphetamine, caffeine (above 12 mcg/ml), ephedrine, certain β_2 agonists
- *Narcotics:* e.g. diamorphone, pethidine, methadone
- *Anabolic agents:* e.g. nandrolone, DHEA, testosterone
- *Diuretics:* e.g. furosemide, bendrofluazide
- *Peptide and glycoprotein hormones and analogues:* e.g. growth hormone, erythropoietin

Classes of drugs subjected to restrictions
- *Alcohol and marijuana* – restricted in certain sports.
- *Local anaesthetics* – local or intra-articular injection only (provide written notification of administration for relevant medical authority).
- *Corticosteroids:* topical, inhaled, or local/intra-articular injection only (provide written notification of administration for relevant medical authority).
- *β-blockers:* restricted in certain sports.

Drugs for pain relief: Generally paracetamol, all NSAIDs and codeine are allowed for pain relief. Stronger opiods and drugs containing caffeine are banned. If in doubt, check on the drug information line (below) before prescribing.

UK Sport produces a card giving more detailed information. Available from UK Sport, 40 Bernard Street, London WCA 1ST ☎ 020 7211 5100 🖥 www.uksport.gov.uk (information resources). Status of a particular medicine may be checked on the Drug Information Line ☎ 0800 528 0004 or 🖥 www.uksport.gov.uk/did

Chapter 4

Diagnosis and management of adult musculoskeletal problems

69

Neck problems

> ⚠ **Neck trauma:** Any significant cervical trauma requires neck immobilization with a hard collar and referral to A&E for cervical spine x-rays to exclude vertebral fracture or instability that could threaten the spinal cord.

Neck pain is common (lifetime incidence 50%) and contributes to 2% of GP consultations. Prevalence is highest in middle age. Most neck pain is acute and self-limiting (within days/weeks) but 1:3 patients presenting to the GP with neck pain have symptoms lasting >6mo. or recurring pain.

History
- Pain: onset, site, radiation, aggravating and relieving factors, timing
- Stiffness: timing – continuous? Worse in the mornings?
- Deformity: e.g. torticollis. Onset, changes
- Neurological symptoms: numbness, paraesthesiae, weakness
- Other symptoms: weight loss, bowel/bladder dysfunction, sweats

ⓘ Pain is often poorly localized and neck problems commonly present with shoulder pain and/or headache (cervicogenic headache) so diagnosis may be difficult.

Examination
- **Look**
  - Posture
  - Deformity e.g. torticollis, asymmetry of scapulae
  - Arms and hands: wasting, fasciculation? Leg weakness?
- **Feel**
  - Tenderness? Midline tenderness may be due to supraspinous damage following a whiplash injury. Paraspinal tenderness ± spasm radiating into the trapezius is common with cervical spondylosis.
  - Warmth? Suggests acute inflammation or infection.
  - Crepitation: common with cervical spondylosis.
- **Move/Measure:** *Normal ranges:*
  - Flexion/extension: 130° total range.
  - Lateral flexion: 45° in each direction from a neutral position.
  - Rotation: 80° in each direction from a neutral position.
- **Neurology:** Weakness in the upper limbs in a segmental distribution, with loss of dermatomal sensation and altered reflexes indicates a root lesion (Table 4.1) . If cervical cord compression is suspected, examine the lower limbs looking for upgoing planters and hyperreflexia.

Cervical spondylosis
- Degenerative disease of the cervical spine can cause pain but minor changes are normal (especially >40y.) and usually asymptomatic.
- Pain is usually intermittent and related to activity.
- Examination reveals ↓ neck mobility. Severe degeneration can cause nerve root signs.
- Treat with analgesia.

X-ray only if conservative measures fail, troublesome pain, nerve root signs or the patient has psoriasis (?psoriatic arthropathy).

Table 4.1 Neurology associated with cervical nerve root entrapment

Root	Sensory changes	Motor weakness	Reflex changes
C5	Lateral arm	Shoulder abduction/ flexion Elbow flexion	Biceps
C6	Lateral forearm Thumb Index finger	Elbow flexion Wrist extension	Biceps Supinator
C7	Middle finger	Elbow extension Wrist flexion Finger extension	Triceps
C8	Medial side of lower forearm Ring and little fingers	Finger flexion	None
T1	Medial side of upper forearm	Finger abduction/ adduction	None

GP Notes: Don't forget other causes of neck pain: e.g.

- Shoulder problems (📖 p.80)
- Temporomandibular joint problems
- Ankylosing spondylitis and psoriatic spondylitis (📖 pp.138–140)
- Rheumatoid arthritis (📖 p.130)
- Polymyalgia rheumatica (📖 p.148)
- Calcium pyrophosphate dihydrate disease (pseudogout – 📖 p.142)
- Diffuse idiopathic skeletal hyperostosis (DISH)
- Fibromyalgia (📖 p.154)
- Myeloma
- Metastatic disease
- Infection – e.g. Staphylococcal, TB
- Osteomalacia (📖 p.118)

Advice for patients: Further information for patients

Arthritis Research Campaign (ARC): ☎ 0870 850 5000
🖥 www.arc.org.uk

Nerve root irritation or entrapment: Secondary to degeneration, vertebral displacement or collapse, disc prolapse, local tumour or abscess. Causes neck stiffness, pain in arms or fingers, ↓ reflexes, sensory loss and ↓ power. The level of entrapment can usually be determined clinically (📖 pp.6–9). In order of frequency:

- $C_{5/6}$ – affects thumb sensation and biceps muscle power
- C_7/T_1 – affects little finger sensation and flexor carpi ulnaris power
- $C_{6/7}$ – affects middle finger sensation, triceps reflex may be absent and latissimus dorsi weak
- $C_{4/5}$ – gives shoulder pain and upper arm weakness

Management
- Analgesia ± cervical collar.
- X-ray cervical spine – lateral or oblique views.
- Refer for physiotherapy.
- Refer for further investigations (e.g. MRI) if conservative management fails and there is objective evidence of a root lesion.

> ⚠ **Refer urgently to neurosurgery** if there are signs of spinal cord compression:
> - Root pain and lower motor neurone signs at the level of the lesion *and*
> - Spastic weakness, brisk reflexes, up-going plantars, loss of co-ordination and sensation below the lesion.

Spasmodic torticollis (wry neck): Common. Sudden onset, painful, stiff neck due to spasm of trapezius and sternocleidomastoid muscles. Self-limiting. Heat, gentle mobilization, muscle relaxants and analgesia can speed recovery. A cervical collar may help in the short term but can prolong symptoms. Often caused by poor posture e.g. computer/seating position; sleeping without adequate neck support; carrying heavy uneven loads.

Cervical rib: Congenital condition – C_7 vertebra costal process enlargement. Usually asymptomatic but can cause thoracic outlet compression, leading to hand or forearm pain, weakness or numbness and thenar or hypothenar wasting. Radial pulse may be weak.

Management: X-ray of thoracic outlet may show cervical rib – but symptoms are sometimes due to fibrous bands that are not seen on x-ray. Refer to upper limb orthopaedic surgeon for further assessment.

Whiplash injuries: Neck pain due to stretching or tearing of cervical muscles and ligaments due to sudden extension of neck – often due to a RTA. Pain and ↓ neck mobility typically starts several hours or days after injury. Pain may radiate to shoulders, arms and head.

Management:
- Examine carefully to exclude bony tenderness requiring x-ray.
- Treat with analgesia and early mobilization – collar may help initially but avoid long-term use.
- Recovery is often slow and 40% patients suffer long-lasting symptoms. As a general rule of thumb, the quicker the symptoms develop, the longer they will take to disappear.
- Psychological problems and medico-legal issues can affect progress.

Advice for patients: Self-help for neck pain and whiplash

In the first 24 hours: An ice-pack applied to the neck will help to relieve inflammation. Bags of frozen peas make particularly good ice-packs because they mould to the body.
- First wrap the ice-pack in a towel or cloth to avoid direct contact between the skin and the ice.
- Lie in bed with your head resting on a pillow and the ice-pack between the pillow and your neck for 20 minutes at a time.

Painkillers: Try normal painkillers you can buy from the chemist such as paracetamol or ibuprofen. Take them regularly for the first few days and then as needed. If these don't help, consult your GP.

Exercise: Research shows that people recover more quickly from whiplash and neck pain if they keep mobile. Here are some exercises you could try.

1. Stand against a door or a wall with your head facing forward and move your eyes so you look towards the 2, 4, 8 and 10 o'clock positions. Repeat this a few times.
2. Beach ball/soft ball exercises: Place a ball between the wall and your forehead and then try to move it around on the wall in circles or figures of eights. Repeat the exercise, this time placing the ball between the back of the head and the wall.
3. Next, take a step forward and perform the following movements.
    - Keep your face straight and upright. Draw your head back and the chin down slightly – rather like a sergeant major.
    - Draw your chin in towards your neck and bend your head carefully forward until you are looking at the floor. Return to the starting position. Repeat slowly 5 times.
    - Bend your head backwards far enough to look at the ceiling. Return to the starting position.
    - Tilt your head sideways, so the right ear is near the right shoulder. If possible try to keep your eyes looking at a fixed point straight ahead. Return to the starting position.
    - Repeat this action with the head tilted to the other side.
    - Turn your head as if trying to look backwards over your shoulder, first to the left 5 times, and then to the right 5 times. Imagine following a horizontal line on the wall at eye level.
4. Lastly, loosen up your shoulders. Shrug as far up as you easily can and then downwards further than normal. Bring your shoulders to the front as if you are trying to get them to meet at the middle, then brace them right back, pulling your shoulder blades together. Repeat this manoeuvre 5 times slowly.

⚠ If any of the exercises makes the pain worse or causes dizziness, stop that exercise. If symptoms are not improving within 2 weeks, go to see your doctor to discuss if a physiotherapy referral would be worthwhile.

73

Low back pain

- *Acute low back pain:* New episode of low back pain of <6wk. duration. Common – lifetime prevalence 58%.
- *Chronic low back pain:* Back pain lasting >3mo. If present >1y. → poor prognosis.

Causes of back pain: Table 4.2

Prevention of back pain
- Regular exercise
- Optimize weight
- Advice re posture, working environment and lifting techniques
- Correct uneven leg length of >2–3cm measured from pubis to medial malleolus

History
- Circumstances of pain – history of injury; duration
- Nature and severity of pain – pain/stiffness mainly at rest or at night, easing with movement, suggests inflammation e.g. discitis, spondyloarthropathy
- Associated symptoms e.g. numbness, weakness, bowel or bladder symptoms
- PMH – past illnesses (e.g. carcinoma), previous back problems
- Exclude pain not coming from the back (e.g. GI or GU pain)

Examination
- Look for deformity e.g. kyphosis (typical of AS), loss of lumbar lordosis (common in acute mechanical back pain), scoliosis.
- Palpate lumbar vertebrae for tenderness or step deformity. Palpate for muscle spasm.
- Assess flexion, extension, lateral flexion and rotation of the back whilst standing.
- Ask to lie down – this gives a good indication of how severe symptoms are.
- In lower limbs look for muscle wasting and check power, sensory loss and reflexes (knee jerk and ankle jerk). Assess straight leg raise (SLR) – sciatica is present if SLR on one side elicits back/buttock pain (usually ipsilateral but can be either side) compared to SLR on the other side.

⚠ 'Red flags'
- <20 or >55y.
- Non-mechanical pain – particularly pain that worsens when supine or night-time pain
- Thoracic pain
- History of carcinoma – consider spinal cord compression. If suspected refer as an emergency to oncology
- HIV
- Immune suppression
- IV drug use
- Taking steroids
- Unwell
- Weight ↓
- Widespread neurology
- Structural deformity

The 'PQRST' rule (see next page) is reproduced with permission from the *ABC of rheumatology*, BMJ Publishing.

Table 4.2 Causes of back pain: age suggests the most likely cause

Age (y.)	Causes	
15–30	• Postural • Mechanical • Prolapsed disc • Trauma	• Fracture • Ankylosing spondylosis • Spondylolisthesis • Pregnancy
30–50	• Postural • Degenerative joint disease • Prolapsed disc	• Discitis • Spondyloarthropathies
>50	• Postural • Degenerative • Osteoporotic collapse • Paget's disease	• Malignancy (lung, breast, prostate, thyroid, kidney) • Myeloma
Other causes	• Referred pain • Spinal stenosis	• Cauda equina tumours • Spinal infection

Table 4.3 Neurology associated with lumbosacral nerve root entrapment

Root	Sensory changes	Motor weakness	Reflex changes
L2	Front of thigh	Hip flexion/adduction	None
L3	Inner thigh	Knee extension	Knee
L4	Inner shin	Knee extension Foot dorsiflexion	Knee
L5	Outer shin Dorsum of foot	Knee flexion Foot inversion Big toe dorsiflexion	None
S1	Lateral side of foot/sole	Knee flexion Foot plantarflexion	Ankle

75

GP Notes: Questions to ask when assessing low back pain

P What factors Provoke and Palliate the pain?
Q What type or Quality of pain is it?
R Does the pain Radiate anywhere?
S How Severe is the pain and are there any Systemic symptoms?
T At what Times is the pain at its best/worst?

Advice for patients: Information and support for patients

- HMSO: *The back book* ISBN 001 702 0788
- Arthritis Research Campaign (ARC): ☎ 0870 850 5000
  🖳 www.arc.org.uk

Management of acute pain in the GP surgery
- *Triage according to history and examination*
- *Don't x-ray routinely:* x-rays require a high radiation dose and +ve findings are rare. *Exceptions:* young (<25y.) – x-ray SI joints to exclude ankylosing spondylitis; elderly – to exclude vertebral collapse/malignancy; history of trauma; 'red flag' signs; no improvement in >6wk.

For patients who don't require immediate referral:
- *Explain the likely natural history* of the pain and advise to avoid bed rest and try to maintain normal activities (↓ chance of chronic pain).
- *Prescribe analgesia* e.g. paracetamol ± NSAIDs.
- *Consider referral for physiotherapy, chiropractic or osteopathy:* Refer patients with nerve root irritation or simple backache not returning to normal activities by 6wk. for back exercises (if available locally) or physiotherapy, chiropractic or osteopathy. Refer sooner if in a lot of pain. Do not refer if there is any possible serious pathology.

Risk factors for developing chronic pain/long-term disability
- Belief that pain and activity are harmful
- Sickness behaviours such as extended rest
- Social withdrawal
- Emotional problems e.g. low/negative mood, depression, anxiety, stress
- Problems with claims or compensation or time off work
- Overprotective family *or* lack of support
- Inappropriate expectations of treatment e.g. low expectations of active participation in treatment

Screening questionnaires (e.g. *New Zealand screening questionnaire for psychosocial barriers to recovery*, available at 🖳 www.nzgg.org.nz) can be helpful in identifying individuals at high risk of developing chronic problems at an early stage.

Management of chronic pain: Aim to help patients accept and cope with pain and to lead as full a life as possible. Education, exercise and psychological approaches may ↓ disability.
- *Exclude spinal pathology and lesions amenable to surgery* e.g. disc protrusion and spondylolisthesis.
- *Consider referral to a pain clinic.*
- *Analgesics* can help sleep disturbance but are of limited benefit if used regularly long term. Reserve for exacerbations.
- *Tricyclic antidepressants* e.g. amitriptyline 25–75mg nocte may be helpful.
- *Other approaches:* Back supports (e.g. corsets or belts); heel raises (to correct uneven leg length) and TENS are sometimes helpful.

Further information
PRODIGY: *Guidance on lower back pain* 🖳 www.prodigy.nhs.uk

Figure 4.1 Triage of acute back pain

Acute back pain

Possible fracture?
History of major trauma (or minor trauma if known osteoporosis)? — Yes → Plain x-ray → Refer immediately if fracture detected, otherwise follow up in 10 d. On follow-up, if fracture still suspected, or multiple sites of pain, consider bone scan and referral

No ↓

Possible cauda equina syndrome or rapidly progressive neurological deficit?
On History
• Saddle anaesthesia or
• Sphincter dysfunction (bladder or bowel)
On examination
• Severe or progressive lower limb neurological deficit/major motor weakness
• Unexpected laxity of the anal sphincter, or
• Perianal/perineal sensory loss
— Yes → Immediate referral

No ↓

Possible serious pathology?
Any 'red flag' signs (🕮 p.74)? — Yes → Check FBC, ESR (↑ in metastases, myeloma, discitis and often ankylolsing spondylitis)
Check Ca^{2+}; phosphate and alkaline phosphatase (↑ in Paget's and tumours)
Arrange lumbar spine and pelvis x-ray

No ↓

↓ Refer if any abnormalities on testing or if not resolving in <4wk.

Nerve root pain?
• Pain radiates to the foot or toes
• Unilateral leg pain is worse than the low back pain
• Numbness or parasthesia present in the same direction as the pain
• SLR reproduces leg pain
• Localized neurological signs (e.g. absent ankle jerk)
— Yes → Specialist referral not needed in first 4wk. assuming signs of resolution

No ↓

Simple backache?
• Age 20–55y.
• Well
• Mechanical pain in lumbosacral area, buttock or thighs
No symptoms/signs inflammatory disease
— Yes → Specialist referral not needed

77

Advice for patients: Self-help back exercises

1. Stretching exercise

NB. Upper knee should be directly above lower knee

1. Back stretch (stretches back muscles) Lie on your back, hands above your head. Bend your knees and, keeping your feet on the floor, roll your knees to one side, slowly. Stay on one side for 10 seconds. **Repeat 3 times each side**.

2. Deep lunge (stretches muscles in front of thigh and abdomen) Kneel on one knee, the other foot in front. Lift the knee up; keep looking forwards. Hold for 5 seconds and **repeat 3 times each side**.

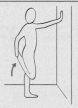

3. One-leg stand–front (stretches front thigh) Steady yourself with one hand on something for support. Bend one leg up behind you. Hold your foot for 10 seconds and **repeat 3 times each side**.

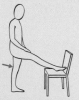

4. One-leg stand–back (stretches muscles at back of leg) Steady yourself, then put one leg, straight, up on a chair. Bend the other knee in to stretch the hamstrings. **Repeat 3 times each side**.

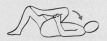

5. Knee to chest (stretches muscles of bottom–gluteals) Lie on your back. Bring one knee up and pull it gently into your chest for 5 seconds. **Repeat for up to 5 times each side**.

2. Strength, stamina and stabilizing exercises

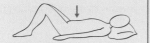

1. Pelvic tilt Lie down with your knees bent. Tighten your stomach muscles, flattening your back against the floor. Hold for 5 seconds. **Repeat 5 times**.

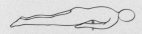

2. Stomach tone ('transverse tummy') Lie on your front with your arms by your side, head on one side. Pull in your stomach muscles, centred around your tummy button. Hold for 5 seconds. **Repeat 3 times**. Build up to 10 seconds and repeat during the day, while walking or standing. Keep breathing during this exercise.

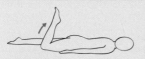

3. Buttock tone (gluteals) Bend one leg up behind you while lying on your front. Then lift your bent knee just off the floor. Hold for up to 8 seconds. **Repeat 5 times each side**.

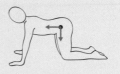

4. Deep stomach muscle tone (stabilizes lolwer back) Kneel on all fours with a small curve in your lower back. Let your stomach relax completely. Pull the lowerpart of your stomach upwards so that you lift your back (without arching it) away from the floor. Hold for 10 seconds. Keep breathing! **Repeat 10 times**.

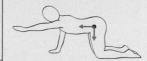

5. Back stabilizer Kneel on all fours with your back straight. Tighten your stomach. Keeping your back in position, raise one arm in front of you and hold for 10 seconds. Try to keep your pelvis level and do not rotate your body. **Repeat 10 times each side**. To progress, try lifting one leg behind you instead of your arm.

79

Exercises on these pages are reproduced with permission of the Arthritis Research Campaign
🖳 www.arc.org.uk

Shoulder problems

> ⚠ Consider pain referred from the neck, cardiac ischaemia and diaphragmatic irritation (gall bladder disease, subphrenic abscess, PE) in all patients presenting with shoulder pain.
>
> If shoulder pain is bilateral, consider polymyalgia rheumatica.

History

- **Pain and stiffness:** Joint pain is felt anteriorly and may radiate down the arm; pain on top of the shoulder suggests acromioclavicular joint problems or cervical spine disorders. Remember pain in the shoulder may be referred from the neck, heart, mediastinum or diaphragm.
- **Deformity:** Swelling of the shoulder; prominence of the acromioclavicular (AC) joint; winging of the scapula.
- **Loss of function:** Difficulty reaching behind back (e.g. doing up bra strap), brushing hair or dressing.

Examination: When the shoulder is in the neutral position, the arm is hanging down with palm facing forwards.

- **Look:** Posture (e.g. arm is held internally rotated in posterior shoulder dislocation); asymmetry; muscle wasting; swelling (large effusions can be seen anteriorly); scars
- **Feel:** Tenderness; warmth; swelling; crepitus
- **Move/measure:** Compare both sides. *Check:*
  - *Range of movement* – Table 4.4
  - *Complex movements* – ask the patient to scratch their opposite scapula in 3 different ways (*scratch test* – ability to do this suggests shoulder joint and tendons are not at fault); hands behind head (external rotation – *capsulitis test*); arm across front of chest to top of opposite shoulder (*scarf test* – AC joint function).
  - *Power* – test for winging of the scapula and deltoid and pectoralis major power. Resist movements of the shoulder – abduction (tests supraspinatus); lateral rotation (tests infraspinatus); medial rotation (tests subscapularis) – check pain and power.

> ### ⚠ Red flags
>
> - Past history of carcinoma
> - Constitutional symptoms e.g. fever, chills or unexplained weight ↓
> - Recent bacterial infection
> - Intravenous drug use
> - Immune suppression
> - Constant worsening rest pain
> - Structural deformity

Causes of a stiff, painful shoulder joint

- Adhesive capsulitis: usually 1° but may be 2° to DM or intrathoracic pathology – 📖 p.82
- Inflammation: inflammatory arthropathy (e.g. RA, psoriatic), infection
- Osteoarthritis – 📖 p.126
- Prolonged immobilization e.g. hemiplegia, strapping after dislocation
- Polymyalgia rheumatica – 📖 p.148

Table 4.4 Normal range of shoulder joint movements

Movement	Test	Normal range
Passive glenohumeral abduction	Ask the patient to flex the elbow. For the right shoulder, stand behind the patient with left hand on the shoulder. Abduct the shoulder with the right hand. Reverse the procedure to test the left shoulder.	90°
Active abduction	Ask the patient to put his hand up, as if pretending to be a bird flapping its wing. Watch to see how the movement is initiated, the range of movement and the arc of painful movement.	180° ❶ initiation is abnormal if there is a ruptured rotator cuff
Active adduction	Adduct the straight arm, carrying the arm in front of the chest as far as it will go.	50°
External rotation	Ask the patient to bend the elbow to 90° and then rotate the arm laterally as far as it will go.	60°
Internal rotation	Ask the patient to put his hand behind his back as far as it will go.	90°
Flexion	Ask the patient to swing the straight arm forwards as far as it will go, like when doing back crawl.	180° (~½ due to glenohumeral joint movement)
Extension	Ask the patient to swing the straight arm backwards as far as it will go, like a soldier marching.	65°

GP Notes: General rules

- Intra-articular disease usually produces painful limitation of movement in all directions.
- Tendonitis produces painful limitation of movement in one plane only.
- Tendon rupture or neurological lesions produce painless weakness.

Rotator cuff injury: The shoulder is the most mobile joint in the body and relies on the musculo-tendinous rotator cuff to maintain stability. Disorders of the rotator cuff account for most shoulder pain.

- *Acute tendonitis:* Often caused by excessive use or trauma in the young (<40y.). Severe pain in the upper arm. Patients hold the arm immobile and are unable to lie on the affected side. Usually starts to resolve spontaneously after a few days. In middle age can be caused by inflammation around calcific deposits – requires steroid injection.
- *Rotator cuff tears:* May accompany subacromial impingement pain (below) and is difficult to diagnose clinically unless the tear is large – suspect if subacromial impingement pain is recurrent. Refer to an upper limb orthopaedic surgeon.
- *Subacromial impingement:* Pain occurs in a limited arc of abduction (60–120° – *painful arc syndrome*) or on internal rotation due to acromial or ligament pressure on a damaged rotator cuff tendon.
  - *Patients <40y.* – associated with glenohumeral instability from generalized connective tissue laxity, or labral injury (see recurrent dislocation below).
  - *Older patients* – often due to chronic rotator cuff tendonitis or functional cuff weakness or tear.

Investigations: X-rays may show calcification of the supraspinatus tendon in acute tendonitis and irregularities/cysts at humeral greater tuberosity if chronic cuff tendonitis.

Treatment: Rest followed by mobilization and physiotherapy, NSAIDs and/or subacromial steroid injection (📖 p.176). If conservative measures fail refer for imaging, arthroscopy and consideration for surgery.

Frozen shoulder (adhesive capsulitis): Overdiagnosed in primary care. Affects patients aged 40–60y. Painful, stiff shoulder with global limitation of movement – notably external rotation. Pain is often worse at night. Cause unknown but ↑ in diabetics, and those with intrathoracic pathology (MI, lung disease) or neck disease.

Management: If not known to be diabetic, check fasting blood glucose. NSAIDs, physiotherapy and local steroid injection can all be helpful. May take >1y. to recover and long-term outcome is uncertain. If restricted movements are slow to return consider orthopaedic referral.

Shoulder OA: Often occurs after a history of trauma. Less common than knee or hip OA. Often associated with crystal-induced inflammation and 2° causes of OA (e.g. gout, haemochromatosis). Imaging for synovitis (USS/MRI) is important to rule out disease that may benefit from steroid injection. Shoulder replacement may be considered in severe cases.

Acromioclavicular joint problems: Pain on the top of the shoulder or in the suprascapular area suggests a problem with the acromioclavicular (AC) joint or neck. AC joint pain is usually due to trauma or OA – joint tenderness and pain are present on palpation and passive horizontal adduction. *Management:* NSAIDs ± local steroid injection.

Advice for patients: Self-help exercises

Range of motion: Stand up and lean over so you're facing the floor. Let the bad arm dangle straight down. Draw circles in the air with the arm. Start with small circles, and then draw bigger ones. Repeat 5–10 times per day. If you have pain doing this, stop and try again later.

Rotator cuff strengthening: Use a piece of thick elastic for these exercises. Stand next to a closed door with a door knob. Tie a loop in one end of the elastic and tie the other end around the door knob. Stand sideways on to the door, bend your arm at a 90° angle and grab the loop. Pull the band across your tummy. At first, do one set of 10 excercises. Try to increase the number of sets as your shoulder pain lessens. These exercises should be done every day.

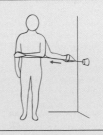

Upper extremity strengthening: Lie on your right side with your left arm at your side. With a weight (e.g. can of baked beans) in your left hand and your forearm across your tummy, raise your forearm. Keep your elbow near your side.

Further information for patients
Arthritis Research Campaign (ARC): ☎ 0870 850 5000
🖳 www.arc.org.uk

Rupture long head of biceps: Discomfort in arm on lifting and a feeling of 'something going'. A lump appears in the body of biceps muscle on elbow flexion. May be associated with other shoulder pathology. *Management:* Exclude distal rupture of the tendon at the elbow. Reassure. No treatment necessary.

Shoulder dislocation: Usually due to fall on arm or shoulder – anterior dislocation is most common.

- Shoulder contour is lost (flattering of deltoid) and the head of the humerus is seen as an anterior bulge.
- Axillary nerve may be damaged → absent sensation on a patch below the shoulder.
- Occasionally immediate reduction is possible (i.e. on the sports field) but beware of concurrent fractures – refer to A&E for X-ray and reduction.
- In young patients ~30% have recurrent dislocations afterwards due to labral tears.
- Dislocation is associated with rotator cuff tear in ~25% of elderly patients.

Recurrent dislocation: Usually anterior and follows trauma – but 5% recurrent dislocations are in teenagers with no history of trauma but general joint laxity. Refer for specialist physiotherapy and consideration of surgery.

Fractured clavicle: Common injury (5% all fractures). Occurs in neonates as a birth injury. In children/adults usually results from a fall onto an outstretched arm. 80% fractures are in the middle $1/3$; 15% the lateral $1/3$ and 5% the medial $1/3$. Refer to A&E for confirmation of diagnosis and fracture clinic follow-up. Treatment is with sling support and analgesia. Most heal well. Complications include pneumothorax, malunion, and nerve/vessel damage.

Elbow problems

History
- **Pain and stiffness:** Joint pain is diffuse; pain well localized over the medial or lateral epicondyles may be due to tendonitis.
- **Deformity:** Swelling? Nodules? Structural deformity?
- **Loss of function:** May be limitation of flexion, extension, pronation and/or supination. This can affect function e.g. causing difficulty eating (can't get hand to mouth) or with personal care.
- **Neurology:** Numbness and paraesthesiae distal to the elbow, particularly in the ulnar nerve distribution.

Examination
- **Look:** Carrying angle (~11° for a ♂; 13° for a ♀). Effusion may be visible either side of the olecranon. A discrete swelling over the olecranon could be RA nodule, gouty tophus, olecranon bursa or other nodule. Check for muscle wasting.
- **Feel:** Tenderness? Swellings? Warmth? If indicated test neurology and check pulses distal to the elbow.
- **Move:** Active and passive movements. Compare both sides. Normal range is from 0° in full extension to 145° in full flexion. Check pronation/supination. Normal range is 75° and 80° respectively.

Tennis elbow and golfer's elbow (epicondylitis)
- *Tennis elbow:* tenderness over the lateral epicondyle and lateral elbow pain on resisted wrist extension.
- *Golfer's elbow:* tenderness over the medial epicondyle and medial elbow pain on resisted wrist pronation.

Common extensor tendon inflammation at the epicondyle. *Cause:* Repeated strain. *Management:* Stop trigger movements if possible. Often settles with time ± NSAIDs. Recovery is speeded by local steroid injection (📖 p.174). Physiotherapy may help, as may an epicondylar clasp.

Dislocated elbow: Usually due to fall on outstretched hand with flexed elbow. Ulna is displaced backwards, elbow is swollen and held in fixed flexion. May have associated fracture. Refer to A&E for reduction.

Pulled elbow: 📖 p.32

Olecranon bursitis: Traumatic bursitis due to repeated pressure on the elbow. Pain and swelling over olecranon. Aspirate fluid from bursa – send for microscopy to exclude sepsis and gout (request polarized light microscopy). Fluid may reaccumulate – if sepsis has been excluded, inject hydrocortisone to help it settle. Refer septic bursitis for drainage.

Ulnar neuritis: Narrowing of the ulnar grove (from OA, RA or post-fracture) causes pressure on ulnar nerve → ulnar neuropathy. Clumsiness with the hand is often the first symptom, then weakness ± wasting of hand muscles innervated by the ulnar nerve and ↓ sensation in the little finger and medial ½ of the ring finger. Rule out metabolic and autoimmune causes of a mononeuritis and refer for consideration of surgical decompression ± nerve conduction studies if entrapment is likely.

Advice for patients: Self-help exercises for tennis elbow

1. Wrist flexor stretch
- Keeping your injured elbow straight, grasp that hand with your other hand and slowly bend the wrist back (palm facing away) until a stretch is felt.
- Hold for 10 seconds.
- Repeat 5 times.

2. Wrist extensor stretch
- Keeping your injured elbow straight, grasp that hand with your other hand and slowly bend the wrist down (palm facing you) until a stretch is felt.
- Hold for 10 seconds.
- Repeat 5 times.

3. Biceps curls
- Support your injured arm with the opposite hand and bend your elbow to full flexion.
- Slowly straighten your arm and repeat 30 times.
- When you can do this easily, start adding some weight into the injured hand e.g. a tin of beans.

Wrist and hand problems

History
Wrist:
- *Pain/stiffness:* Pain is often well localised in the wrist. 5 conditions are associated with point tenderness:
  - De Quervain's disease
  - Old scaphoid fracture
  - Carpometacarpal osteoarthritis
  - Kienbock's disease (avascular necrosis of the lunate)
  - Tenosynovitis of the extensors.

  Wrist pain may also be associated with osteoarthritis, rheumatoid arthritis and ganglia. Carpal tunnel syndrome is associated with pain in the hand.
- *Deformity:* May be swelling of tendon sheaths or wrist. Bony deformity is a late feature of arthritis or secondary to trauma.
- *Function:* Ask about weakness and numbness in the hand.

Hand:
- *Pain/stiffness:* Pain from the hand is felt in the fingers and/or palm. A diffuse ache may be referred from the neck, shoulder or mediastinum.
- *Deformity:* May occur acutely e.g. due to tendon rupture or slowly due to bone or joint pathology. The pattern and symmetry of joint involvement can be diagnostic.
- *Function:* Good hand function is essential for everyday tasks e.g. turning keys, doing buttons up, writing. Ask about limitations.

Examination
Wrist:

- *Look:* Symmetry left vs. right; swelling; deformity (ulnar deviation, volar subluxation; rheumatoid nodules; ganglia); muscle wasting in forearm and hand
- *Feel:* Temperature; nature of any swellings; tenderness of the radiocarpal joint, midcarpal joint or distal radio-ulnar joint
- *Move/measure:* Range of movement (normal range – extension >75°, flexion >75°, pronation >75° from the vertical, supination >80° from the vertical); crepitation?
- *Neurology:* Check for ulnar and median nerve function.

Hand:
- *Look:* Posture of the hand; swellings (rheumatoid nodules; Heberden's and Bouchard's nodes; ganglions; tophi); nail signs e.g. pitting of psoriasis; scars; deformity (mallet finger; swan-neck deformity; Boutonniere deformity; Dupytrens contracture); ulnar deviation. If there is joint disease, note distribution and whether it is symmetrical.
- *Feel:* Temperature; condition of the skin e.g. dryness, sweating; nature of swellings; muscle bulk e.g. small muscles of the hand; tenderness
- *Move/measure:* Ask the patient to make a fist, spread his fingers out and then test each individual joint. Then test opposition, pinch grip, key grip, palmar grasp of ball and practical tasks e.g. picking up a coin.

GP Notes: For all hand injuries

Check for

Nerve injury: Can occur due to trauma or lacerations of the hand or wrist. Examine sensory and motor function. Always ensure no other structures are damaged before suturing skin wounds. Refer all nerve injuries for specialist assessment and management – surgery can improve the outcome considerably. Intensive hand physiotherapy is important to regain function. Types of nerve injury:

- *Neurapraxia:* temporary loss of nerve conduction – often caused by pressure causing ischaemia.
- *Axonotmesis:* damage to the nerve fibre but the nerve tube is intact – the chance of successful nerve regrowth and a good recovery is high.
- *Neurotmesis:* Divided nerve – lack of guidance to the regrowing fibrils gives less chance of a good recovery and a neuroma may develop.

Median nerve damage: The median nerve controls grasp. Damage causes inability to lift the thumb out of the plane of the palm (abductor pollicus brevis failure) and loss of sensation over the lateral side of the hand.

Ulnar nerve damage: Injury distal to the wrist causes a claw hand deformity, loss of abduction/adduction of the fingers and sensory loss over the little finger and a variable area of the ring finger.

Radial nerve damage: The radial nerve opens the fist – injury produces wrist-drop and variable sensory loss including the dorsal aspect of the root of the thumb.

Tendon injury: Can occur due to attrition or lacerations of the hand or wrist. Examine hand function. Always ensure no other structures are damaged before suturing skin wounds. Extensor or flexor tendons can be affected. Refer – primary surgical repair is usually the treatment of choice.

Vascular injury: Can occur due to trauma or lacerations of the hand or wrist. Check perfusion and temperature of fingers and examine pulses. Always ensure no other structures are damaged before suturing skin wounds. Refer all vascular injuries for specialist assessment and management.

89

Advice for patients: Further information for patients

Arthritis Research Campaign (ARC): ☎ 0870 850 5000
🖳 www.arc.org.uk

Tenosynovitis: Inflammation of the tendon sheath – often due to unaccustomed activity (e.g. gardening). May affect extensor or flexor tendons. Pain is often worse in the morning. Presents with swelling and tenderness over the tendon sheath and pain on using the tendon.

Management: Rest and NSAIDs. If not settling an injection of steroid into the tendon sheath can help.

De Quervain tenosynovitis: Tenosynovitis of thumb extensor and abductor tendon sheaths causing pain over radial styloid and on forced adduction and flexion of the thumb.

Management: Thumb splint, local steroid injection or surgery as a last resort.

Ganglion: Smooth, firm, painless swelling – usually around the wrist. No treatment is needed unless causing local problems. May resolve spontaneously; can be drained (large-bore needle)/excised, but often recurs.

Work-related upper limb pain: Work-related pain in the arm ± wrist e.g. related to keyboard use. Overuse syndrome. Often termed repetitive strain injury (RSI). Diagnosis of exclusion – no physical signs. Exclude other conditions e.g. carpal tunnel syndrome (CTS), tennis elbow.

Management: Reassure – condition is curable, continue work but avoid the aggravating activity, liaise with work to ensure evaluation of workstation ergonomics. Gradually reintroduce activity. Physiotherapy may help. Explore psychological and work-related issues. A multidisciplinary approach is needed.

Existence of RSI has been challenged – rigorous assessment often reveals undiagnosed causes. A country's compensation system has a great effect on the reporting of RSI.

Carpal tunnel syndrome: Pain in the radial 3½ digits of the hand ± numbness, pins and needles and thenar wasting. Due to compression of the median nerve as it passes under the flexor retinaculum (Figure 4.2). Worse at night. Symptoms are improved by shaking the wrist. *Associations:* Pregnancy, hypothyroidism, obesity and carpal arthritis.

Investigations
- Phalen's test: hyperflexion of wrist for 1 min. triggers symptoms (Figure 4.3).
- Tinel's test: tapping over the carpal tunnel causes paraesthesiae.
- Nerve conduction studies if diagnosis is in doubt.

Management
- Night splints may help.
- Carpal tunnel steroid injection (📖 p.174).
- Surgery to divide the flexor retinaculum is curative in mild/moderate disease.

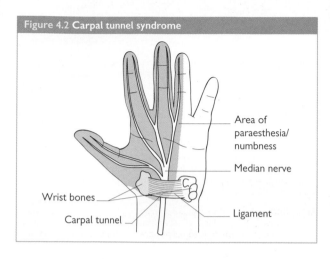

Figure 4.2 **Carpal tunnel syndrome**

Area of paraesthesia/numbness

Median nerve

Wrist bones

Carpal tunnel

Ligament

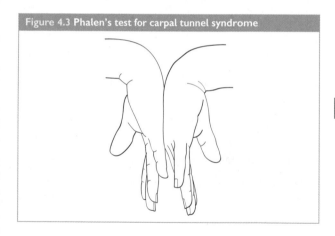

Figure 4.3 **Phalen's test for carpal tunnel syndrome**

GP Notes:

Tenosynovitis and repetitive strain injury are both notifiable industrial diseases – 📖 p.192.

Colles' fracture: Most commonly due to a fall onto an outstretched hand in an elderly woman. Pain and swelling of the wrist ('dinner-fork' deformity). Refer any suspected fracture for x-ray.

⚠ Always consider assessment and treatment for osteoporosis in all men and women >50y. who have had a Colles' fracture – 📖 p.122.

Scaphoid fracture: Caused by falling onto an outstretched hand. Pain, swelling and tenderness in the anatomical snuff box. Symptoms may be mild and a fracture is easily missed – refer all suspect cases for scaphoid view x-rays. If x-ray is inconclusive and pain continues, repeat 2wk. later – bone scan can help if still –ve. Non-union and avascular necrosis of the proximal fragment is a potential complication, which can lead to long-term problems of arthritis and pain.

Kienbock's disease: The lunate bone develops patchy necrosis after acute or chronic injury. Patient is usually a young adult complaining of aching and stiffness of 1 wrist. *Examination:* Tenderness in the centre of the back of the wrist ± limitation of wrist extension. X-ray is normal at first but later shows ↑ density of the lunate ± deformity. Refer for orthopaedic opinion.

Osteoarthritis in the hand
- Heberden's nodes: swellings of DIP joints. No treatment needed.
- Bouchard's nodes: swellings of PIP joints. No treatment needed.
- First carpometacarpal OA: pain and swelling at the base of the thumb. Thumb becomes stiff. A splint or steroid injection can be helpful. If pain persists surgery may help.

Dupuytren contracture: Palmar fascia contracts so that the fingers (typically the right 5th finger) cannot extend. *Prevalence:* 10% of men >65y. (more if family history). Less common in women. *Associations:* Smoking; alcohol; heavy manual labour; trauma; DM; phenytoin; Peyronie's disease; AIDS. *Management:* Often simple reassurance suffices. Ultimately surgery to release the contracture may be required.

Fractured fingers: Refer all suspected fractures for x-ray ± reduction.
- *Fractured metacarpal* (fractured 5th metacarpal is most common): normally heals if immobilized in a wool and crepe bandage for 10d.
- *Fracture proximal phalanx:* normally associated with a rotation deformity and may require open surgical reduction and fixation.
- *Fracture middle phalanx:* often can be manipulated into position and splinted by strapping to the next finger.
- *Terminal phalanx:* usually a crush fracture – protect with a mallet splint.

Trigger finger: Nodules on the tendon can occur spontaneously and in RA and DM. Most common in ring and middle fingers. The nodule can be palpated moving with the tendon. Pain and triggering (the finger in fixed flexion needs to be flicked straight by the other hand) occur because the nodule jams in the tendon sheath. *Management:* Local steroid injection or surgery.

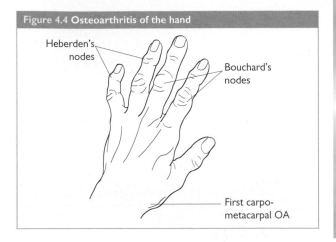

Figure 4.4 Osteoarthritis of the hand

Heberden's nodes

Bouchard's nodes

First carpo-metacarpal OA

Mallet finger: The finger tip droops due to avulsion of the extensor tendon attachment to the terminal phalanx. Refer for x-ray. *Management:* A plastic splint which holds the terminal phalanx in extension is worn for 6wk. to help union (must not be removed). Arthrodesis may be needed if healing doesn't occur.

Gamekeeper thumb: Forced thumb abduction causes rupture of the ulnar collateral ligament. Can occur on wringing a pheasant's neck, hence the name, or, more commonly, by catching the thumb in the matting on a dry ski slope. The thumb is very painful and pincer grip weak. Refer – open surgical repair is the most effective treatment.

Nail injuries:
- *Avulsed nail:* Protect the nail bed of an avulsed nail with soft paraffin and gauze, check tetanus status and give antibiotic prophylaxis (e.g. flucloxacillin 250mg qds for 5d.). Partially avulsed nails need removing under ring block to exclude an underlying nail bed injury – the nail is replaced to act as a splint to the nail matrix.
- *Subungual haematoma:* A blow to the finger can cause bleeding under the nail – very painful due to pressure build-up. Relieve by trephining a hole through the nail using a 19-gauge needle (no force required, just twist the needle as it rests vertically on the nail) or a heated point (e.g. of a paper clip or cautery instrument). Of benefit up to 2d. after injury.

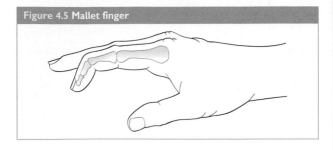

Figure 4.5 Mallet finger

Hip problems

History
- **Pain/stiffness:** Pain on walking? Pain at rest? Hip joint pain is usually felt in the groin (Table 4.5). Referred pain is often felt in the knee.
- **Function:** Hip disease results in ↓ walking distance, difficulty climbing stairs and getting out of low chairs.

Examination
- **Look:** Watch the patient walk – hip disease → limp or waddling gait.
- **Feel:** Joint tenderness is found just distal to the midpoint of the inguinal ligament.
- **Move:** Passive movement with the patient lying down on his back. Check range of movement – pain reproduced on movement? crepitus?
  - *Flexion:* Flex the patient's knee and move the thigh towards the chest.
  - *Rotation:* Flex the hip and knee. With one hand on the knee and the other on the foot, move the foot medially to test for external rotation then laterally to test for internal rotation (normal range ~45° in both directions).
  - *Abduction and adduction:* Move the leg away from the midline (abduction – normal range ~50°) then towards the midline (adduction – normal range ~45°).
  - *Extension:* Ask the patient to turn onto his stomach. Lift each leg in turn. Normal range is ~30°.
- **Measure:** Hip disease is often associated with shortening of the affected leg.
  - True leg length: Anterior superior iliac spine → medial malleolus
  - Apparent leg length: Umbilicus → medial malleolus
- **Trendelenburg test:** Ask the patient to stand on one leg and lift the foot on the contralateral side off the ground (Figure 4.6). Place your fingers on the anterior superior iliac spines. If the pelvis sags on the unsupported side – positive Trendelenburg sign. The hip on which the patient is standing is painful (resulting in gluteal inhibition) or has a weak or mechanically disadvantaged gluteus medius (subluxation/dislocation of the hip, coax vara, slipped epiphysis, muscle weakness e.g. due to a root lesion, polio or a muscle wasting disease).

> Trendelenburg test gives a false +ve in 10% of cases.

Groin pain in athletes: *Consider:*
- Conjoint tendon pathology (Gilmour's groin)
- Symphysitis (footballers notably) *and*
- Adductor tendonitis.

Liaise with a sports medicine physician or physiotherapist early.

Table 4.5 Causes of pain around the hip

Pain	Causes
Buttock pain	PMR, sacroilitis, vascular insufficiency, referred from back
Groin pain	Hip joint disease (OA, RA, Paget's, osteomalacia), fracture, osteitis pubis, hernia, psoas abscess
Lateral thigh pain	Trochanteric bursitis, referred pain from back, enthesitis (spondyloarthropathies), gluteus medius tear, meralgia paraesthetica, fascia lata syndrome

Figure 4.6 The Trendelenburg test

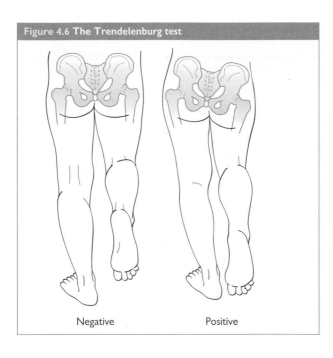

Negative   Positive

Osteoarthritis of the hip: Major cause of hip pain and disability. Incidence ↑ with age; ♂≈♀.

Predisposing factors: Past hip disease (e.g. Perthes) or trauma; unequal leg length.

Presentation: Pain may be diffuse and felt in hip region, thigh or knee. Relieved by rest in early stages of disease. Signs: ↓ internal rotation and abduction of hip with pain at extremes of movement; antalgic gait; eventually fixed flexion of the hip. Investigation: X-ray may confirm diagnosis but is often not needed. There is poor correlation between x-ray changes and pain felt.

Management: Analgesia (e.g. regular paracetamol, NSAIDs), education, weight ↓, exercise, correction of unequal leg length. Walking stick ± shock-absorbing shoe insoles can help. Consider referral for physiotherapy (muscle strengthening exercises may ↓ pain) or to orthopaedics for consideration of hip resurfacing or replacement.

Total hip replacement: >90% achieve good result. Most last 10–15y. *Post-op care:* Risk of dislocation in the 1st 6wk. – advise to avoid crossing legs; take care with transfers; use a walking stick; no driving for 6wk. Physiotherapy is usually arranged via secondary care.

Malignancy: Hip and pelvis are common sites for 2° malignancy. Pain is severe and unremitting, day and night. Often accompanied by ↓ weight. X-ray may show no abnormalities or reveal lytic or sclerotic deposits. Bone scan is diagnostic but may miss myeloma. Depending on clinical circumstances either refer for specialist advice (oncologist, radiotherapist) or palliative care. Treat with analgesia meanwhile. High risk of pathological fracture.

Hip fracture: Common amongst the elderly – carries high morbidity and mortality (≈25%). ♀>♂. Usually occurs through the neck of the femur. *Risk factors:* Maternal hip fracture, osteoporosis, unsteadiness, sedative medication, poor eyesight and polypharmacy. There may be a history of a fall but not always. Suspect in any patient who is elderly or has risk factors for osteoporosis (📖 p.120) who is 'off legs'. Occasionally patients may still be able to weight bear with difficulty. *Signs:* External rotation, and shortening of the leg.

Management: Refer urgently to A&E for x-ray.

Hip dislocation: Occurs in front-seat passengers in car accidents as the knee strikes the dashboard. Reduction under anaesthetic is required. High risk of 2° degenerative change.

Greater trochanter pain (trochanteric bursitis): Can mimic ± coexist with hip OA. May be associated with muscle weakness around the hip. *Diagnosis:* Point tenderness over the greater trochanter.

Management: Consider local steroid injection if trochanteric bursitis is likely, though most cases are due to referred back pain. Refer to physiotherapy for exercises to strengthen hip musculature to prevent recurrence or for treatment of back problems if causing the pain.

Advice for patients: General advice for patients with hip osteoarthritis

- Sit in a partially reclined position when relaxing.
- Stand with weight equally distributed between both legs.
- Lift and carry weight close to the body.
- Sleep on the unaffected side with a large pillow between the knees.
- Keep your weight down.
- Exercise regularly e.g. swimming with crawl kick (legs kept straight).
- Avoid extremes of hip motion.
- Minimize jarring and high-impact activities e.g. contact sports like football or 'stop-and-go' sports like tennis.

Self-help exercises

🟡 It may help to have a warm bath or to apply a heat pad to the affected hip before doing these exercises.

Knee–chest pulls: Lie on your back. Bend your hip and knee to 90°. Hold your upper shin and gently pull your knee towards your chest. Hold this position for 5 seconds and then relax back to 90°. Repeat 15–20 times every day.

Figure of four stretch: Still lying on your back, put your foot beside your other knee. Gently rock your knee outwards. Repeat 15–20 times each day. The higher the foot is raised the greater the stretch.

Straight-leg raises (strengthening the hip flexors): Still lying on your back, bend one leg. Keep the opposite leg straight and raise it 5–10cm (3–4 inches) off the bed and hold it there for 5 seconds. Do this 15–20 times with each leg every day.

Leg extensions (strengthening the gluteals): Turn over onto your tummy. Raise one leg 5–10cm (3–4 inches) up off the bed and hold it there for 5 seconds. Repeat 15–20 times for each leg every day.

🟡 If any of these exercises causes pain, stop and consult your doctor or physiotherapist before doing that exercise again.

⚠ These exercises are NOT suitable for patients who have had a hip replacement.

Further information for patients

Arthritis Research Campaign (ARC): ☎ 0870 850 5000
🖳 www.arc.org.uk

Fascia lata syndrome: Inflammation of the fascia lata causing pain in the lateral thigh. Often due to overuse or weak musculature around the hip. Treatment is with rest ± referral to physiotherapy.

Hip infection: Presents with hip pain, ↓ weight, night sweats and rigors. Be aware of infection in patients with RA, hip prosthesis or immunocompromise. Refer for investigation. X-rays are often unhelpful – bone scan is non – specific.

Management: Admit for ultrasound-guided drainage, bed rest and IV antibiotics.

Avascular necrosis: May present with hip pain. Have a high level of suspicion in patients with risk factors – SLE, sickle cell disease, high alcohol consumption, pregnancy or corticosteroids. X-ray or bone scan may confirm diagnosis but MRI is most sensitive. Specialist management is needed. Usually progresses to cause OA.

Advice for patients: Further information for patients

Arthritis Research Campaign (ARC): ☎ 0870 850 5000
🖥 www.arc.org.uk

Knee problems

History
- **Trauma:** History of injury – ask about degree and direction of force.
- **Pain/stiffness:** Attempt to distinguish well-localised mechanical pain and diffuse inflammatory/degenerative pain.
- **Deformity:** Swelling? If injury, time of onset of swelling in relation to history (immediate effusion suggests haemarthrosis; post-traumatic effusions appear later). Knock knees or bow legs?
- **Function:**
  - Does the knee problem prevent any activities? How far can the patient walk? Can they manage stairs?
  - Does the knee click? If so, when?
  - Does the knee lock? If so, what position does the knee lock in? What provokes locking and how is it relieved?
  - Does the knee give way? If so, when (e.g. when going downstairs, when walking on uneven ground)?

Examination: Always compare the 2 knees.

ⓘ Knee pain can be referred from the hip so examine the hip as well.

- **Look:** Watch the patient walk. Look at the knees whilst standing – ?varus/valgus deformity. Ask the patient to lie down. Note quadriceps wasting, scars, skin changes, swelling and deformity. A space under the knee viewed laterally suggests a fixed flexion deformity. With legs extended, lift both feet off the bed to demonstrate hyperextension.
- **Feel:**
  - Feel the quadriceps for wasting and palpate the knee for warmth.
  - Check the joint line, collateral ligaments, tibial tubercle and femoral epicondyles for tenderness.
  - Palpate the popliteal fossa for a baker's cyst.
  - Check for an effusion (Table 4.6, 📖 p.105).
  - Test for patellofemoral lesions by sliding the patella sideways across the underlying femoral condyles.
- **Move:** With the patient lying on their back check:
  - *Active and passive movement:* Check full range of movement (full extension – 135° flexion). Pain reproduced on movement? Crepitus?
  - *Medial and lateral collateral ligaments:* Holding the leg just above the knee with one hand, and foot with the other, flex the hip slightly and with a slightly flexed knee, apply an abducting and then adducting force to the foot whilst holding the knee still (Figure 4.7). If the knee opens up (>5° movement is abnormal) there is collateral and/or cruciate ligament damage.
  - *Cruciate ligaments:* Flex the knee to 80–90° and sit on the end of the foot to fix it in place. Place both hands around the top of the calf. Attempt to sharply pull the tibia forwards to test anterior cruciate laxity and push it backwards to test posterior cruciate laxity (Figure 4.8). More than a small degree of movement suggests significant laxity.
- **Measure:** Quadriceps diameter 18cm up from the joint line in adults.

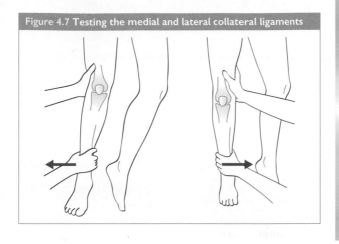

Figure 4.7 Testing the medial and lateral collateral ligaments

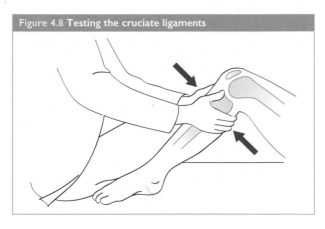

Figure 4.8 Testing the cruciate ligaments

Non-traumatic knee effusion: *Common causes:*
- Gout
- Calcium pyrophosphate dihydrate disease (pseudogout)
- Spondyloarthropathies (includes reactive arthritis)
- RA

Investigation:
- Blood: FBC, ESR, rheumatoid factor, anti-nuclear antibody, LFTs, bone biochemistry and thyroid function tests.
- Drain effusion (or refer to rheumatology to drain) and send fluid for polarized light miscroscopy (for crystals) and microbiology (?infection).

Management:
- If no infection inject with long-acting steroid, immobilize and advise no weight bearing for 48h.
- Refer to rheumatology.

Osteoarthritis of the knee: Very common. X-ray evidence of OA is even commoner. *Treatment:* Education; glucosamine; analgesia (paracetamol ± NSAIDs); exercise (refer to physiotherapy ± exercise programme – self-help exercises 📖 p.107 and 109). Suggest using a walking stick. Steroid injection can be helpful in some patients. If pain and disability are severe refer to orthopaedics for consideration of total knee replacement.

Total knee replacement Very successful procedure → ↓ pain and ↑ mobility. 95% of prostheses last 10y.

Infection of the knee joint: Most commonly infected joint. *Signs:* Hot, red, swollen, painful knee. *Differential diagnosis:* Reiter's disease, gout, pseudogout, traumatic effusion, RA. If infection is suspected refer as an emergency to rheumatology or orthopaedics for investigation.

104

⚠ Don't give antibiotics until the joint has been aspirated.

Growing pains: 📖 p.30

Chondromalacia patellae: Common in teenage girls. Pain on walking up or down stairs or on prolonged sitting. *Signs:* Pain on stressing the undersurface of the patella. Arthroscopy (indicated only in severe cases) reveals degenerative cartilage on the posterior surface of the patella. *Management:* Analgesia + physiotherapy (vastus medialis strengthening relieves pain in 80%). For persistent cases, exclude spondyloarthropathy (enthesitis pain – 📖 p.138) and refer to orthopaedics for arthroscopy.

Osgood-Schlatter disease: Seen in athletic teenagers. Pain and tenderness ± swelling over the tibial tubercle. X-rays not required. *Management:* Avoid aggravating activities. Usually settles over a few months. If not settling refer to orthopaedics or rheumatology for further assessment.

Hypermobility: Is associated with knee pain, especially if associated patellar subluxation. A FH of hypermobility is common. Pain may be aggravated by exercise. Extremely hypermobile individuals may have a hereditary connective tissue disorder (e.g. Ehlers-Danlos syndrome) and may suffer from premature OA. Refer for specialist rheumatology advice.

Table 4.6 Testing for a knee effusion

Test	Procedure
Cross-fluctuation	Easiest test for large effusions. Compress the suprapatellar pouch with the left hand, Straddle the front of the joint with the right hand below the patella. Squeeze each hand alternately. If fluid is present, a fluid impulse is transmitted across the joint.
Patellar tap	Can confirm a medium/large effusion. Squeeze excess fluid from the suprapatellar pouch with your index finger and thumb. Start ~15cm above the knee and advance the thumb and index finger distally to the level of the upper border of the patella. With the tips of the fingers of the free hand, tap the patella sharply downwards towards the bed. Positive if the patella sinks and stops with a tap as it contacts the femur. False negative if the effusion is small or very tense.
Bulge sign	Can detect a small effusion. Empty the suprapatellar bursa by squeezing distally from ~15 cm above the patella. Empty the medial compartment of the joint by pressing on the side of the joint with the free hand. Then lift this hand away and sharply compress the lateral side (Figure 4.9). Positive if a ripple is seen on the flattened, medial surface. False negative if effusion is tense.

Figure 4.9 The bulge sign

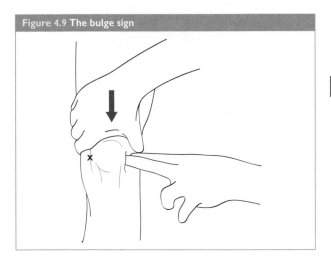

Patellar dislocation: Lateral dislocation of the patella and tearing of the medial capsule and quadriceps can occur due to trauma. More common in young people and in joint hypermobility syndrome. Patient is in pain and unable to flex knee. Refer via A&E or orthopaedics for reduction.

Recurrent subluxation of the patella: Medial knee pain + knee 'gives way' due to lateral subluxation of the patella. Most common in girls with valgus knees. *Associations:* Familial, hypermobility, high-riding patella. *Signs:* ↑ lateral patella movement and +ve apprehension test (pain and reflex contraction of quadriceps on lateral patella pressure).

Management: Refer to physiotherapy for vastus medialis exercises. If that is unhelpful, refer to rheumatology to exclude a hereditary connective tissue disorder and/or to orthopaedics for consideration of lateral retinacular release.

Bipartite patella: Detected on X-ray. Usually asymptomatic incidental finding but can cause pain due to excessive mobility of a patella fragment. If troublesome refer for fragment excision.

Patella tendonitis: Small tear in the patella tendon causes pain. Most commonly seen in athletes. Differential includes inferior patellar pole enthesitis (spondylarthropathies), fat-pad syndrome, anterior cartilage lesion and bursitis. Diagnosis is with USS. *Treatment:* Rest, NSAIDs ± steroid injection around (not into) the tendon.

Bursitis: Prepatella bursitis (housemaid's knee) is associated with excessive kneeling. Vicar's knee (infrapatella bursitis) is associated with more upright kneeling.

Management: Avoid aggravating activity, aspirate ± steroid injection (↓ recurrence). If clinically infected refer to orthopaedics for drainage and antibiotics.

Baker's cyst: Popliteal cyst (herniation of joint synovium) can cause swelling and discomfort behind the knee. Usually caused by a degenerative knee. Rupture may result in pain and swelling in the calf mimicking DVT. Treat underlying knee synovitis. Surgical cyst removal may be necessary if persistent problems.

Iliotibial tract syndrome: Pain due to inflammation of the synovium under the iliotibial tract from rubbing of the tract on the lateral femoral condyle. Seen in runners.

Management: Rest, NSAIDs, specialist physiotherapy ± steroid injection.

Osteochondritis dissecans: Necrosis of articular cartilage and underlying bone. Can cause loose body formation. Cause unknown. Seen in young adults → pain after exercise and intermittent knee swelling ± locking. X-ray shows cartilage damage. Predisposes to arthritis. Refer for expert management.

Advice for patients: Self-help knee exercises 1

Start with 'low-impact exercises' (non-weight-bearing i.e. sitting or lying on the floor, sofa or bed) and build toward weight-bearing exercises and functional activities, e.g. walking.

Sit on the floor, sofa or bed with your legs outstretched. Keeping your foot on the floor (or sofa/bed), slowly bend one knee until you feel the knee being confortably stretched without hurting; hold for 3–4 seconds. Straighten your leg as far as you can; hold for 5 seconds. Repeat until you have done 10 bends. Repeat the exercise with the other leg.

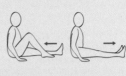

Sitting on the floor, sofa or bed with your legs outstretched, place a rolled-up towel under one knee. Push down on the towel as if straightening your knee, then pull your toes and foot towards you so that you feel your calf muscles stretch and so that your heel lifts off the floor (or sofa/bed). Hold for 5 seconds, relax for 5 seconds, then repeat until you have done 10 contractions. Repeat the exercise with the other leg.

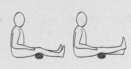

If you have a set of pedals or static exercise bike, adjust the pedals so that your knee is straight at the lowest position of a revolution. Cycle without any resistance at a comfortable pace for 2 minutes, increasing the time as you improve. Once you can do that easily, if you have a static exercise bike with variable resistance, over a period of weeks increase the resistance you are pedalling against to improve your strength and stamina.

Most days try and get out for a walk, gradually increasing the distance you walk over several weeks. Don't be worried about using a stick or having frequent rests to relieve the stress on your joints.

More knee self-help exercises: 📖 p.109

Further informtion for patients

Arthritis Research Campaign (ARC) ☎ 0870 850 5000
🖳 www.arc.org.uk

Collateral ligament injury: Common in contact sports. Causes knee effusion if severe ± tenderness over the injured ligament. Collateral ligaments provide lateral stability to the knee. Normally there is <5° of movement; if >5° the ligament may be ruptured.

Management: Rest, knee support, analgesia. Refer to orthopaedics if rupture suspected.

Cruciate ligament injury: Cruciate ligaments provide anterior/posterior knee stability.
- *Anterior cruciate tears:* Occur due to a blow to the back of tibia ± rotation when foot is fixed on the ground. *Signs:* Effusion and +ve draw test (with the patient supine with foot fixed and knee at 90°, apply pressure to pull the tibia forward – it should be stable – test is +ve if the tibia moves forward on the femur).
- *Posterior cruciate tears:* Caused e.g. when the knee hits the dashboard in car accidents. Reverse draw test is +ve (with patient supine and knee at 90°, apply pressure to push tibia backwards – it should be stable – test is +ve if the tibia moves backward on the femur).

Management: Refer to orthopaedics. Assessment can be difficult – refer if unsure. Plaster cast and then physiotherapy helps most (60%) but some require reconstructive surgery – consider urgent referral if keen sportsperson.

Meniscal lesions: Twisting with the knee flexed can cause medial (bucket handle) meniscal tears and adduction with internal rotation can cause lateral cartilage tears. *Symptoms/signs:*
- Locking of the knee: extension is limited due to cartilage fragment lodging between the condyles.
- Giving way of the knee.
- Tender joint line.
- +ve McMurray test: rotation of the tibia on the femur with flexed knee followed by knee extension causes pain and a click as the trapped cartilage fragment is released – reliability of this test is debated.

Management: Refer for MRI ± arthroscopy. Treated by removal of the torn meniscal fragment.

Meniscal cysts: Pain + swelling over the joint line due to a meniscal tear. Lateral cysts are more common than medial. The knee may click and give way. Refer for arthroscopy – removal of damaged meniscus relieves pain.

Loose bodies in the knee: May result in locking of the knee joint in any direction of movement and/or effusion. *Causes:* OA, chip fractures, osteochondritis dissecans, synovial chondromatosis. If problematic refer for removal.

Shin splints: Exercise-related shin pain may be due to a stress fracture of the tibia, compartment syndrome or periostitis. Fractures are not always seen on x-ray – bone scan is more sensitive and shows periostitis.

Management: Rest and analgesia. Consider referral to sports physiotherapist.

Advice for patients: Self-help knee exercises 2

Exercises to strengthen your thigh muscles – start by trying to do these exercises twice a week, then build up gradually so you are doing them every other day and then every day

Sitting on a chair, cross one leg behind the other. Push forward with the back leg as if to straighten it, but prevent this happening by pushing back with the front leg. Push as hard as possible for 5 seconds, then relax completely for 3 seconds, repeat, and after 6 contractions rest for 1 minute. Repeat this procedure until you have done 4 sets of 6 contractions (24 contractions in total). Repeat the exercise with the other leg in front.

Sitting on a chair, fold your arms, slowly stand up and then slowly sit down, ensuring each 'sit–stand' is slow and controlled. Do 'sit–stands' for 1 minute, count the number you do and write this in a notebook. Over a period of weeks try to increase the number of 'sit–stands' you can do in 1 minute. As you improve, try the 'sit–stands' from progressively lower chairs or the bottom two steps of a staircase.

Place your right foot on the bottom step of the stairs, using the banisters for support. Keeping this leg on the step, step up and down with the left leg. Count and record the number of step-ups you perform in 1 minute. Rest for 1 minute, then repeat the exercise keeping your left leg on the step. As the number of step-ups you can perform per minute increases, increase the height of the step (ensuring you are stable and safe) to a maximum of about 45cm (18 inches).

Holding onto a stable object (e.g. chair or table), squat down slowly, keeping your back straight and bending both knees, then straighten your knees. Do not squat down too far for the first couple of weeks. As you feel improvement and the exercise gets easier you can squat a little further, but only until your knees are bent to 90° – never squat down fully.

Tie the elastic inner tube of a bicycle tyre to an immovable object (e.g. the leg of your bed or the chair you will sit on) and loop it around your right foot with your knee bent. Sitting on the chair or the edge of your bed, slowly straighten your knee, stretching out the band. Hold your leg straight for 5 seconds, then control the band as it slowly bends your knee back to the starting position. Do this for about 1–2 minutes. Repeat the exercise with the band around your left foot. As you improve, you can do the exercise for longer and/or the resistance can be increased by making the loop smaller or using a stiffer band.

Further information for patients

Arthritis Research Campaign (ARC) ☎ 0870 850 5000 🖳 www.arc.org.uk

Ankle and foot problems

History
- **Trauma:** History of injury. History of ↑ activity e.g. walking or running further than the patient is used to. Is there a feeling of instability?
- **Pain/stiffness:** Relation to weight bearing; localized or diffuse?
- **Deformity:** Swelling, bunions, flat feet, congenital foot abnormalities e.g. past history of talipes. Does the patient have any problems getting shoes to fit comfortably? Do shoes wear in odd places?
- **Function:** Does the problem prevent any activities? How far can the patient walk? Does they need a walking aid? Can they manage stairs?

Examination: Compare one foot with the other:
- **Look:** Watch the patient walk. Ask them to stand and walk on tiptoe. Look at the foot with the patient sitting with their foot on your lap or on an examination couch. Are there any swellings or obvious deformities e.g. drop foot, pes cavus, bunions, hammer or mallet toes, talipes? Look at the colour of the foot and skin/nails – are there any callosities or corns? Are there signs of psoriasis on the nails? Check shoes for abnormal patterns of wear (wear is normally under the ball of the foot medially and posterolaterally at the heel).
- **Feel:** Is there any tenderness? Palpate any swellings. Check pulses and skin temperature.
- **Move:** Assess active and passive movements of the ankle, subtalar, mid-tarsal and toe joints systematically. Is there any pain on movement? Is the power normal? Is there any crepitus?
  - *Ankle flexion/extension:* Normal range from the neutral point at right angles to t
  - he leg is 55° plantar flexion and 15° dorsiflexion.
  - *Ankle ligaments:* Grasp the heel and forcibly invert the foot. Opening up of the ankle joint with this procedure implies damage to the lateral ligament. Dorsiflexion causes pain as the tibia is displaced laterally if there is damage to the inferior tibio-fibular ligament.
  - *Eversion and inversion of the foot.*
  - *Mobility of metatarsal heads:* Hold the heel with one hand; move the foot with the other hand in dorsal and plantar directions, assessing mobility of the 1st, 4th and 5th metatarsal heads. Squeeze the metatarsals to detect tender inflammation common in early RA or Morton's neuroma.
  - *Flexion and extension of the toes:* Normal range of flexion of the big toe is 40° and it has 65° extension.
- **Neurology:** Check sensation if patient reports any loss of sensation.

Causes of foot pain
Forefoot: Forefoot pathology (e.g. pes cavus/planus), stress fracture, RA, DM, gout, OA, paralytic deformity, post-traumatic syndrome, nerve root pathology, tarsal nerve compression, Morton's neuroma.

Heel:
- *Within the heel:* Arthritis of the subtalar joint, osteomyelitis, tumours, Paget's disease
- *Behind the heel:* Ruptured Achilles tendon, Achilles tendinitis
- *Under the heel:* Tender heel pad, plantar faciitis, plantar calcaneal bursitis

Twisting of the ankle resulting in pain and swelling is a very common injury. Foot injuries are also common. It can be difficult to distinguish between a sprain and a fracture. The Ottawa rules ↓ need for x-ray by ¼ .

Ottawa rules for ankle and foot x-ray

Ankle injury
Refer for an ankle X-ray if there is pain in the malleolar area AND
- bone tenderness at the posterior tip of the lateral malleolus, or
- bone tenderness at the posterior tip of the medial malleolus, or
- patient is unable to weight bear at the time of the injury and when seen.

Foot injury
Refer for a foot X-ray if there is pain in the midfoot AND
- bone tenderness at the 5th metatarsal base, or
- bone tenderness at the navicular, or
- patient is unable to weight bear at the time of injury and when seen.

Otherwise diagnose a sprain: Treat sprains with rest, ice, compression, elevation and analgesia (paracetamol ± NSAIDs). If severe (or the patient is an athlete), refer to physiotherapy.

Osteochondritis: 📖 p.35

Foot drop: Patients trip frequently or walk with a high-stepping gait. On examination patients are unable to walk on their heels and cannot dorsiflex their foot. Check ankle jerk. *Causes:*
- Common peroneal palsy e.g. due to trauma – normal ankle jerk
- Sciatica – ankle jerk absent
- L4, L5 root lesion – ankle jerk may be absent
- Peripheral motor neuropathy e.g. alcoholic – ankle jerk weak or absent
- Distal myopathy – ankle jerk weak or absent
- Motor neurone disease – ↑ ankle jerk

Achilles tendonitis: Inflammation of the Achilles tendon may be related to overuse or a spondylarthropathy. Presents as a painful local swelling of the tendon.

Management: Rest, NSAIDs, heel padding, physiotherapy. Steroid injection may help (never inject into the tendon). If persistent refer to rheumatology.

Ruptured Achilles tendon: Presents with a sudden pain in the back of the ankle during activity (felt as a 'kick'). The patient walks with a limp. There is some plantar flexion, but the patient cannot raise the affected heel from the floor when standing on tip toe. A 'gap' can usually be felt in the tendon.

Management: Refer immediately for consideration of repair. The alternative is immobilization in plaster with the foot plantar flexed.

Further information:
Bandolier *Ruptured Achilles tendons – systematic review* (2002) 🖥 www.jr2.ox.ac.uk/bandolier/band103/b103-5.html

Tender heel pad: Dull throbbing pain under the heel. Develops over a few months after heel trauma. May be due to plantar fasciitis, bursitis or tendonitis.

Management: Rest and heel padding. Refer to physiotherapy – ultrasound treatment can help. Blind steroid injections into the fat pad are not recommended. In persistent cases refer to rheumatology.

Plantar fasciitis/bursitis: Common cause of inferior heel pain especially amongst runners. Pain is worst when taking the first few steps after getting out of bed. Usually unilateral and generally settles in <6wk.

Management: Advise shoes with arch support (e.g. trainers), soft heels and heel padding. Achilles tendon stretching exercises can help (opposite), NSAIDs and steroid injection are also helpful. In persistent cases refer to rheumatology.

Flat feet (pes planus): Low medial arch. Normal in young children (📖 p.34). Painless flat foot in which the arch is restored on standing on tiptoe ('flexible' foot needs no treatment. If painful may be helped by analgesia, exercises or insoles. For severe pain, hind foot fusion is an option. Refer if the arch does not restore on tiptoeing ('rigid' foot).

Advice for patients: Plantar fasciitis self-help exercises

Routine stretching is very important to healing plantar fasciitis. Most of those affected by plantar fasciitis have decreased flexibility and tight Achilles tendons.

Towel stretch: Sit on the floor with your legs stretching out in front of you. Loop a towel around the top of the injured foot. Slowly pull the towel towards you, keeping your body straight. Hold for 15 to 30 saeconds then relax – **repeat 10 times**.

Calf/Achilles Stretch: Stand facing a wall place your hands on the wall chest high. Move the injured heel back and with the foot flat on the floor. Move the other leg forward and slowly lean toward the wall until you feel a stretch through the calf, hold and repeat.

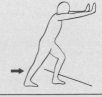

Stair Stretch: Stand on a step on the balls for your feet, hold the rail or wall for balance. Slowly lower the heel of the injured foot to stretch the arch of your foot.

Toe Stretch: Sit on the floor with knee bent. Pull the toes back on the injured foot until stretch across the arch is felt. Hold and repeat.

Frozen can roll: Roll your bare injured foot back and forth from the tip of the toes to the heel over a frozen juice can. This is a good exercise after activity because not only stretches the plantar fascia but provides cold therapy to the injured area.

Pes cavus: High foot arches may be idiopathic, due to polio, spina bifida or other neurological conditions. Toes may claw.

Management: Padding under metatarsal heads relieves pressure. Operative treatment — soft tissue release or arthrodesis straightens toes. Can lead to tarsal bone OA, causing pain — refer for fusion.

Metatarsalgia (forefoot pain): May be due to synovitis stress fracture, sesamoid fracture, injury or ↑ pressure on the metatarsal heads due to mechanical dysfunction (e.g. in RA). Treat with insoles and padding under the MT heads. Surgery may be helpful in RA — discuss with rheumatologist.

Morton's metatarsalgia (interdigital neuroma): Pain due to entrapment of the interdigital nerve between the 3rd/4th metatarsal heads. *Symptoms:* Gradual onset of sudden attacks of pain or paraesthesia during walking.

Management: Steroid injection and advice re footwear may help. Some need surgical excision of the neuroma.

Toe fracture: Often due to dropping a heavy weight onto the toe. Does not need treatment — strapping to the adjacent toe may ↓ pain.

Hammer and claw toes
- *Hammer toes:* Extended MTP joint, hyperflexed PIP joint and extended DIP joint. Most common in 2nd toes.
- *Claw toes:* Extended MTP joint, flexion at PIP and DIP joints. Due to imbalance of extensors and flexors (e.g. after polio).

If causing pain or difficulty with walking/ footwear, refer for surgery.

Hallux valgus (bunion): Lateral deviation of the big toe at MTP joint exacerbated by wearing pointed shoes ± high heels. A bunion develops where the MTP joint rubs on footwear. Arthritis at the MTP joint is common. Bunion pads can help but severe deformity requires surgery.

Hallus rigidus: Arthritis at 1st MTP joint causes a stiff painful big toe. Refer severe cases to podiatrist or orthotist for offloading or custom-made rocker bottom foot orthoses. If pain is persistent, refer for surgical fusion.

Ingrowing toe nail: Most common in the big toe. Ill-fitting shoes and poor nail cutting predispose to the nail growing into the toe skin → pain. The inflamed tissue is prone to infection.

Management: Advise re cutting nails (cut straight with edges beyond the flesh). Refer to podiatry. Treat infection with antibiotics (e.g. flucloxacillin 250–500mg qds). If recurrent problems consider surgery (e.g. wedge resection of the nail).

Figure 4.10 Hammer and claw toes

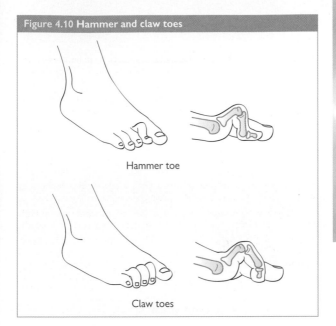

Hammer toe

Claw toes

Advice for patients: Information for patients

British Orthopaedic Foot Surgery Society: 🖥 www.bofss.org.uk

Bone disorders

Paget's disease of bone Accelerated disorganized bone remodelling due to abnormal osteoclast activity. Affects up to 1:10 of the elderly but only a minority are symptomatic. ♂:♀≈3:1.

Presentation:
- Pain: dull ache aggravated by weight bearing – often remains at rest
- Deformity: bowing of weight-bearing bones, especially tibia (sabre), femur and forearm. Usually asymmetrical.
- Frontal bossing of forehead.
- Distinctive changes on x-ray.
- ↑ bone-specific alk phos; normal Ca^{2+}, PO_4, PTH, bone scintigraphy.

Management: Refer to rheumatology. Give analgesia. Bisphosphonates (e.g. risedronate 30mg/d. for 2mo.) ↓ pain and long-term complications.

Complications: Pathological fractures; OA of adjacent joints; high-output CCF; hydrocephalus and/or cranial nerve compression → neurological symptoms e.g. deafness; spinal stenosis; bone sarcoma (10% of those affected >10y.).

Osteomyelitis: Infection of bone. May spread from boils, abscesses or follow surgery. Often no primary site is found. More common in those with DM, impaired immunity sickle cell disease and/or poor living standards. Organisms involved: S. Aureus, Streptococci, E. coli, Salmonella, Proteus and Pseudomonas species, TB.

Signs: Pain, unwillingness to move affected part, warmth, effusions in neighbouring joints, fever and malaise.

Investigation: Blood cultures +ve in 60%, ↑ESR/CRP, ↑WCC.

Management: Refer suspected cases for same-day orthopaedic opinion. Diagnosis is confirmed with imaging e.g. MRI or bone scanning (X-ray changes take a few days to appear). *Treatment:* IV then po antibiotics (≥6wk.) and surgery to drain abscesses.

Complications: Septic arthritis, pathological fracture, deformity of growing bone, chronic infection.

Chronic osteomyelitis: Occurs after delayed or inadequate treatment of acute osteomyelitis. Signs: Pain, fever and discharge of pus from sinuses. It follows a relapsing and remitting course over years. Specialist management is needed.

Bone tumours: Bone is a common site for secondaries from other tumours (e.g. breast, lung, thyroid, kidney and prostate). 1° tumours:
- *Malignant:* All rare – Ewing's sarcoma, osteosarcoma, chondrosacroma.
- *Mixed:* Giant cell tumour (osteoclastoma) is benign histologically but may behave in a malignant way.
- *Benign:* Osteoid osteoma, chondroma and osteochondroma.

Presentation: Aching bone pain, swelling ± pathological fracture.

Management: Refer all bony swellings for X-ray and specialist management – excision, chemotherapy, radiotherapy and reconstruction.

GMS contract

Cancer Indicator 1	The practice can produce a record of all cancer patients diagnosed after 01.04.2003.	5 points	
Cancer Indicator 3	The % of patients with cancer diagnosed within the year with a patient review recorded within 6mo. (in the first year 1.4.2006–31.3.2007) or 3mo. (from 1.4.2007 onwards) of the practice receiving confirmation of diagnosis. This should include an assessment of support needs, if any, and a review of co-ordination arrangements with secondary care.	Up to 6 points	40–90%
Education Indicator 7	The practice has undertaken a minimum of 12 significant event reviews in the past 3y. which include (if these have occurred) 2 new cancer diagnoses.	Total of 4 points for 12 significant event reviews	

GP Notes: Referral guidelines for suspected bone cancer[N]

Refer for immediate x-ray any patient with suspected spontaneous fracture. If the x-ray:
- Indicates possible bone cancer, refer urgently
- Is normal but symptoms persist, follow up and/or request repeat x-ray, bone function tests or referral

Refer urgently if a patient presents with a palpable lump that is:
- >5cm in diameter
- Deep to fascia, fixed or immobile
- A recurrence after previous excision
- Increasing in size
- Painful

❶ If a patient has HIV, consider Kaposi's sarcoma and make an urgent referral if suspected.

Urgently investigate increasing, unexplained or persistent bone pain or tenderness, particularly pain at rest (and especially if not in the joint), or an unexplained limp. In older people metastases, myeloma or lymphoma, as well as sarcoma, should be considered.
Referral of children and young people: 📖 p.31

117

Advice for patients: Information and support for patients

Arthritis Research Campaign (ARC): ☎ 0870 850 5000
🖥 www.arc.org.uk
National Association for the Relief of Paget's Disease:
☎ 0161 799 4646 🖥 www.paget.org.uk

Further information

NICE: *Referral guidelines for suspected cancer – quick reference guide* (2005) 🖥 www.nice.org.uk

Osteomalacia and rickets

Vitamin D deficiency causes rickets in children and osteomalacia in adults. The body needs ~10µg of vitamin D per day to maintain healthy bones. The body makes its own vitamin D when sunlight falls on the skin in the summer months but a diet with adequate vitamin D is needed to maintain the supply in the winter, especially for people who don't get out or for cultural or religious reasons are completely shielded from the sun by their clothing.

Clinical features of rickets

- Bone pain/tenderness: arms, legs, spine, pelvis
- Skeletal deformity: bow legs, pigeon chest (forward projection of the sternum), rachitic rosary (enlarged ends of ribs), asymmetrical/odd-shaped skull due to soft skull bones, spinal deformity (kyphosis, scoliosis), pelvic deformities
- Pathological fracture
- Dental deformities: delayed formation of teeth, holes in enamel, ↑ cavities
- Muscular problems: progressive weakness, ↓ muscle tone, muscle cramps
- Impaired growth → short stature (can be permanent)

Clinical features of osteomalacia

- Bone pain: diffuse – particularly in hips
- Muscle weakness
- Pathological fractures
- Low calcium → perioral numbness, numbness of extremities, hand and feet spasms and/or arrhythmias

Causes and management

Dietary deficiency (<30 nmol/l): Particularly in children with pigmented skin in Northern climes. Give vitamin D and Ca^{2+} supplements.

Age-related deficiency (<30 nmol/l): Vitamin D metabolism deteriorates with age and many >80y. are deficient. Consider giving vitamin D (800iu/d) to all elderly >80y.

Secondary rickets/osteomalacia: Vitamin D deficiency is due to other disease e.g. malabsorption, liver disease, renal tubular disorders or chronic renal failure. Treat underlying cause/supplement Ca^{2+} and vitamin D.

Vitamin D dependent rickets: Rare autosomal recessive disorder resulting in an enzyme deficit in the metabolism of vitamin D. Refer for specialist care. Treated with vitamin D and Ca^{2+} supplements.

Hypophosphataemic rickets (vitamin D resistant rickets): X-linked dominant trait resulting in ↓ proximal renal tubular resorption of phosphate. Parathyroid hormone and vitamin D levels are normal. Specialist management is needed. Treatment is with phosphate replacement ± calcitriol.

Table 4.7 Approximate vitamin D content of common foods

Food	Serving	Vitamin D (µg)
Margarine	10g ($^1/_2$ oz)	0.8
Eggs	1 size 3	1.1
Cheese	60g (2 oz)	0.2
Milk	0.15l ($^1/_4$ pint)	0.05
Butter	10g ($^1/_2$ oz)	0.1
Fortified cereals	30g (1 oz)	0.5
Herring	100g ($3^1/_2$ oz)	16.5
Mackerel	100g ($3^1/_2$ oz)	8
Sardines	100g ($3^1/_2$ oz)	7.5
Tinned tuna	100g ($3^1/_2$ oz)	4
Tinned salmon	100g ($3^1/_2$ oz)	12.5
Kipper	100g ($3^1/_2$ oz)	13.5

Advice for patients: Information and support for patients

Arthritis Research Campaign (ARC): ☎ 0870 850 5000
🖥 www.arc.org.uk

Osteoporosis

Lifetime risk of osteoporotic fracture is 40% in women and 13% in men. The main morbidity and financial costs of osteoporotic fracture relate to hip fracture where incidence ↑ steeply >70y. Treatment aims to prevent fracture.

Definition: Osteoporosis is defined as bone mineral density >2.5 standard deviations (SD) below the young adult mean (T score of −2.5). There is i relative risk of fracture x2–3 for each SD ↓ in BMD.

🚺 Osteopoenia cannot be reliably diagnosed on X-ray – though vertebral fractures may be seen.

Bone mineral density (BMD) measurement: Hip and lumbar spine BMD measurement by Dual energy X-ray absorptionmetry (DEXA) scan can quantify risk of osteoporotic fracture (Figure 4.11).

Check BMD if:
- <75y. and previous fragility fracture
- On long term steroids and <65y.
- If other risk factors for osteoporosis (see below)
- Suggested osteopoenia on X-ray

Follow local referral guidelines until national guidance is available (NICE will publish guidance on primary prevention of osteoporosis in 2007).

The report from the DEXA scan should contain information on fracture risk, management and time interval for re-checking BMD. Generally treatment with a bisphosphonate is started if the T score is ≤ −2.5.

Age as a risk factor for osteoporosis: Risk of osteoporosis and associated fractures ↑ with age as bone mass declines (Figure 4.12).

120

Major age-independent risk factors for osteoporosis
- Glucocorticoid use (📖 p.122)
- Previous fragility fracture (📖 p.122)
- Low BMI (<19 kg/m^2)
- FH of maternal hip fracture aged <75y.
- Untreated premature menopause, prolonged amenorrhoea or ♂ hypogonadism
- Conditions associated with prolonged immobility
- Medical disorder independently associated with bone loss e.g. inflammatory bowel or coeliac disease, chronic liver disease, hyperthyroidism, ankylosing spondylitis, chronic renal failure, type 1 DM, RA

Advice for patients: Information and support

Arthritis Research Campaign ☎ 0870 850 5000
🖥 www.arc.org.uk
National Osteoporosis Society ☎ 0845 450 0230
🖥 www.nos.org.uk

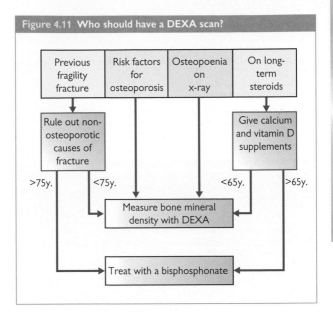

Figure 4.11 **Who should have a DEXA scan?**

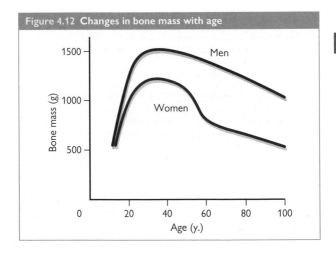

Figure 4.12 **Changes in bone mass with age**

Glucocorticoid use: Steroid use is a risk factor for osteoporosis.
- Minimise steroid dose.
- Advise *all* patients taking any dose of oral steroids to take calcium/vitamin D supplements^G.

In addition: For patients taking oral/high-dose inhaled steroids for >3mo.
- Add a bisphosphonate for patients >65y. *or*
- Refer patients <65y. for DEXA scan and add a bisphosphonate if T score is ≤−1.5.

Previous fragility fracture: Fracture sustained falling from ≤ standing height – includes vertebral collapse (may not be a fall). Previous fracture is a risk for future fracture. Common fractures:
- *Hip:* associated with ↑ mortality
- *Wrist:* Colles'
- *Spine:* Osteoporotic vertebral collapse causes pain, ↓ height and kyphosis. Pain can take 3–6mo. to settle and requires strong analgesia. Calcitonin is useful for pain relief for 3mo. after vertebral fracture if other analgesics are ineffective.

Investigation
- DEXA scan if <75y.
- Exclude other causes of pathological fracture e.g. malignancy, osteomalacia, hyperparathyroidism. Check FBC, ESR, TSH, Cr, bone and liver function tests – all should be normal.
- Consider checking serum paraproteins/urine Bence Jones protein, bone scan and FSH/testosterone/LH (if hormonal status unclear).

Management^N
- If ≥ 75y. treat without DEXA once all non-osteoporotic causes of fracture have been ruled out.
- If 65-74y. treat if DEXA confirms osteoporosis (T score ≤−2.5).
- Treat if <65y. and very low BMD (T score ≤−3) *or* if T score ≤−2.5 and the patient has ≥1 additional age-independent risk factor (📖 p.120).

Lifestyle advice: Provide to all at risk patients.
- *Adequate nutrition:* Approximate amounts of calcium in common foods are listed in Table 4.8 (📖 p.123).and of vitamin D in Table 4.7 (📖 p.119).
  - Maintain body weight so BMI >19kg/m^2.
  - Give Ca^{2+} and/or vitamin D supplements to postmenopausal women with dietary deficiency^C.
  - Supplement with Ca^{2+} (0.5–1g/d.) and vitamin D (800 IU/d.). if on long-term steroids C, >80y., housebound or institutionalized^C.
- *Regular exercise:* Weight-bearing activity >30min/d. ↓ fracture rate^S.
- *Stop smoking[£]* pre-menopause →25% ↓ fracture rate post menopause.
- ↓*alcohol consumption* to <21u/wk. (♂) or <14u/wk. (♀).

Table 4.8 **Approximate calcium content of common foods**		
Food	**Serving**	**Calcium (mg)**
Whole milk	0.2l ($^1/_3$ pint)	220
Semi-skimmed milk	0.2l ($^1/_3$ pint)	230
Hard cheese	30g (1 oz)	190
Cottage cheese	115g (4 oz)	80
Low fat yoghurt	150g (5 oz)	225
Sardines (including bones)	60g (2 oz)	310
Brown or white bread	3 large slices	100
Wholemeal bread	3 large slices	55
Baked beans	115g (4 oz)	60
Boiled cabbage	115g (4 oz)	40

An adult requires ~ 700mg of calcium /day to maintain healthy bones

GP Notes:

Measures to ↓ risk of falls and damage from falling: Falls are one of the biggest risk factors for fracture. Tendency to fall ↑ with age.

- Modify identified hazards or risk factors
- Assess and correct vision, if possible
- Correct postural hypotension – alter medication; consider compression stockings -but many elderly people cannot apply stockings tight enough to be of any use themselves
- Treat other medical conditions e.g. refer to cardiology if arrythmia.
- Review medication and discontinue/alter inappropriate medication
- Remove environmental hazards – arrange bath at a day centre, refer to OT to identify and correct hazards in the home e.g. remove loose carpets, wheeled trolley for use indoors, commode or urine bottle for night time use, moving the bed downstairs etc.
- Refer to OT to identify and correct hazards in the home
- Liaise with other members of the primary healthcare team and social services to provide additional support if needed; refer to local council for 'carephone' or alarm system to call for help if any further falls
- Refer to rehabilitation/physiotherapy to improve confidence after falls and for weight-bearing exercise (focusing on strength and flexibility) and balance training (↓ risk of falls)
- Use of hip protectors.↓ fracture risk in patients at high risk but compliance is a problem[C]

Treatment options

Bisphosphonates: e.g. alendronate 10mg od or 70mg once weekly. ↓ bone loss and fracture rate[C]. Mainstay of treatment and prevention of osteoporosis.

Strontium ranelate: 2g od in water. ↑ formation and ↓ resorption of bone. Use for postmenopausal osteoporosis – particularly when bisphosphonates are contraindicated or not tolerated. ↓ hip/vertebral fracture risk by 36–41%.

Selective oestrogen receptor modulator (SERM) e.g. raloxifene 60mg od -use if bisphosphonates are contraindicated/not tolerated or there is an unsatisfactory response (further fracture and/or ↓ in BMD after ≥1y. treatment) with bisphosphonates

HRT (♀): 📖 p.210. Postpones postmenopausal bone loss and ↓ fractures[C]. Optimum duration of use is uncertain (>5–7y.) but benefit disappears within 5y. of stopping. ↑ breast cancer and cardiovascular risk limits use[R].

> **CSM guidance (2003):**
> - **Premature menopause:** HRT is recommended for the prevention of osteoporosis until women reach 51y.
> - **>51y.:** HRT should **not** be considered 1st line therapy for long-term prevention of osteoporosis. HRT remains an option where other therapies are contraindicated, cannot be tolerated, or if there is a lack of response; risks and benefits should be carefully assessed.

HRT (♂): Supplement testosterone if hyogonadism.

Teriparatide: Most powerful treatment for osteoporosis currently available. Consider referral for consultant initiation if other treatment options are exhausted. Given by daily injection.

Referral: Routinely refer to endocrinology or menopause clinic if:
- Premature menopause (<40y.)
- Unexplained cause of osteoporosis
- Osteoporosis in a man, or
- Problems with management

Further information

NICE 🖥 www.nice.org.uk
- Osteoporosis – secondary prevention (2005)
- Osteoporosis – assessment of fracture risk and prevention in high risk individuals – due for publication in 2006.

National Osteoporosis Society Primary care strategy for osteoporosis and falls (2002) 🖥 www.nos.org.uk

Royal College of Physicians Osteoporosis: Clinical guidelines for prevention and treatment (2003) 🖥 www.rcplondon.ac.uk

CSM Guidance Further advice on safety of HRT (12/2003) 🖥 www.mca.gov.uk

Million Women Study Collaborators. Lancet 2003; 362: 419–427

Women's Health Initiative Study 🖥 www.whi.org

Advice for patients

Frequently asked questions about osteoporosis:

What is osteoporosis? Everybody loses bone as they get older. The amount of body lost varies from person to person. Some people lose so much bone that their bones become fragile and break more easily. Those people have osteoporosis. Osteoporosis is far more common in women than men and usually comes on after the menopause.

Who is at risk of developing osteoporosis? Everyone is at risk of developing osteoporosis as they get older. Some factors make you more at risk. These include having an early menopause or having a period of time when your periods stopped due to an eating disorder, heavy exercise or illness; having a family history of osteoporosis; having a medical history of certain conditions such as an overactive thyroid; or taking steroid tablets for other medical conditions.

Your lifestyle can also put you at risk. You can lower your risk of having thin bones by eating foods which contain calcium and vitamin D or taking supplements, taking plenty of exercise, stopping smoking and cutting down on your alcohol intake.

How is osteoporosis diagnosed? Special X-ray machines do a Dual Energy X-ray Absorptiometry (DEXA) scan which can check your bone density (thickness) and confirm osteoporosis. However, osteoporosis is often first diagnosed when you break a bone.

What are the symptoms and problems of osteoporosis? Osteoporosis usually develops slowly over several years without any symptoms. The major problem associated with osteoporosis is the increased risk of breaking a bone, even after a minor fall. A fractured bone in an older person can be serious. For example, about half the people who have a hip fracture are unable to live independently afterwards.

What are the treatments for osteoporosis? There are a number of medicines which can be prescribed to prevent your osteoporosis getting worse. The most commonly used drugs are the bisphosphonates which include Alendronate, Risedronate and Etidronate.

You can also take measures to help prevent you from falling. This can reduce the chance of you breaking a bone. Check your home for hazards such as loose rugs, slippery floors, and objects you could trip on, and be careful outside in bad conditions, for example if it is wet or icy. If your medicine makes you drowsy, talk to your doctor to see if it can be changed and keep active. If you have had a fall, see your doctor as a 'falls assessment' may help prevent further falls.

Information and support for patients

Arthritis Research Campaign ☎ 0870 850 5000 🖳 www.arc.org.uk
National Osteoporosis Society ☎0845 450 0230 🖳 www.nos.org.uk

Osteoarthritis (OA)

OA is the single most important cause of locomotor disability. It used to be considered as 'wear and tear' of the bone and cartilage of synovial joints but is now recognized as a metabolically active process involving the whole joint i.e. cartilage, bone, synovium, capsule and muscle.

The main reason for patients seeking medical help is pain. The level of pain and disability are greatly influenced by the patient's personality, levels of anxiety, depression and activity and often don't correlate well with clinical signs.

Risk factors

- ↑ age (uncommon <45y.)
- ♀>♂
- ↑ in black and Asian populations
- Genetic predisposition
- Obesity
- Abnormal mechanical loading of joint e.g. instability, previous fracture
- Poor muscle function
- Post-meniscectomy
- Certain occupations e.g. farming.

Symptoms and signs: Joint pain ± stiffness, synovial thickening, deformity, effusion, crepitus, muscle weakness and wasting and ↓ function. Typically exacerbations occur that may last weeks to months. Most commonly affects hip, knee and base of thumb. Nodal OA, with swelling of the distal interphalangeal joints (Heberden's nodes) has a familial tendency.

Investigations: X-rays may show ↓ joint space, cysts and sclerosis in subchondral bone, and osteophytes. Check FBC and ESR if inflammatory arthritis is suspected (normal or mildly ↑ in OA – ESR >30 suggests RA or psoriatic arthritis).

🛈 Exclude other causes of pain i.e. sepsis, bursitis, gout, inflammatory arthritis and fibromyalgia. OA is common and may be a coincidental finding and not the cause of the patient's pain.

Aims of management: *To:*

- Educate the patient
- ↓ pain
- Optimize function
- Minimize progression

Management in primary care: 📖 p.128
Refer

- *To rheumatology* to:
  - Confirm diagnosis if co-existent psoriasis (psoriatic arthritis mimics OA and can be missed by radiologists)
  - Rule out 2° causes of OA (e.g. pseudogout, haemochromatosis) if young OA or odd distribution
  - If joint injection is thought worthwhile but you lack expertise or confidence to do it.
- *To orthopaedics:* if symptoms are severe for joint replacement. Refer as an emergency if you suspect joint sepsis.

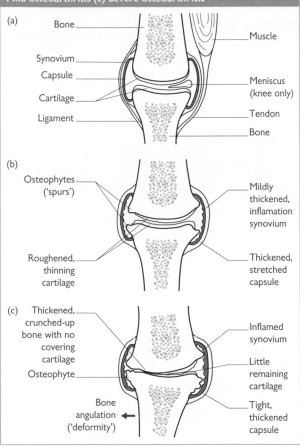

Figure 4.13 **Joint changes in osteoarthritis (a) Normal joint (b) Mild osteoarthritis (c) Severe osteoarthritis**

(a)
Bone
Muscle
Synovium
Capsule
Meniscus (knee only)
Cartilage
Ligament
Tendon
Bone

(b)
Osteophytes ('spurs')
Mildly thickened, inflamation synovium
Roughened, thinning cartilage
Thickened, stretched capsule

(c)
Thickened, crunched-up bone with no covering cartilage
Inflamed synovium
Osteophyte
Little remaining cartilage
Bone angulation ('deformity')
Tight, thickened capsule

Reproduced with permission from Arthritis Research Campaign (ARC) *Osteoarthritis* booklet
☎ 0870 850 5000 ▦ www.arc.org.uk

Management of osteoarthritis in primary care

Information and advice: Give information and advice on all relevant aspects of osteoarthritis and its management. The ARC website (🖳 www.arc.org.uk) has a wide range of information leaflets for patients. Use the whole multidisciplinary team e.g. refer to:
- Physiotherapist for advice on exercises, strapping and splints
- OT for aids
- Chiropodist for foot care and insoles
- Social worker for advice on disability benefits and housing
- Orthopaedic surgeon for assessment for joint replacement if significant disability or night pain.

↓ load on the joint: Weight reduction can ↓ symptoms and may ↓ progression in knee OA. Using a walking stick in the opposite hand to the affected hip and cushioned insoles/shoes (e.g. trainers) can also help.

Exercise and improving muscle strength: ↓ pain and disability e.g. walking (for OA knee), swimming (for OA back and hip but may make neck worse), cycling (for OA knee but may worsen patellofemoral OA). Refer to physiotherapy for advice on exercises, especially isometric exercises for the less mobile.

Pain control:
- Regular paracetamol (1g qds) is effective for many patients.
- NSAIDs are overused and there is no evidence of additional benefit over simple analgesics except in acute exacerbations.
- Topical NSAIDS have fewer side effects than oral NSAIDs
- Systematic review shows they are more effective than placebo in both acute and chronic pain control.[5] Rubefacients and counterirritants (e.g. capsaicin cream) can also be helpful.
- Some patients find local heat or cold soothing.
- Low-dose antidepressants e.g. amitriptyline 10–75mg nocte. (unlicensed) are a useful adjunct, especially for pain causing sleep disturbance.

Aspiration of joint effusions and joint injections: Can help in exacerbations. Some patients respond well to long-acting steroid injections – it may be worth considering a trial of a single treatment. Hyaluronic acid injections improve knee pain in the short/mid term[5] but are associated with short-term ↑ in inflammation.

Glucosamine: 1500mg/d. may improve knee symptoms – consider 3mo. trial of treatment. 🖝 It is controversial whether glucosamine modifies OA progression.

Other complementary therapies: Up to 60% of sufferers from OA are thought to use complementary therapies e.g. copper bracelets, food supplements dietary manipulation (e.g. by eating oily fish and foods rich in vitamins C and E). There is good evidence chiropractic and osteopathy can be helpful for back pain, and acupuncture may help knee pain, but otherwise evidence of effectiveness is scanty. Advise patients to find a reputable practitioner with accredited training who is a member of a recognised professional body and carries professional indemnity insurance.

Psychological factors: Have a major impact on the disability from OA. Education about the disease, and emphasis that it is not progressive in most people, is important. Seek and treat depression and anxiety.

Further information

Bandolier Topical NSAIDS (2003)
🖥 www.jr2.ox.ac.uk/bandolier/band110/b110-6.html

Journal of Family Practice Modawal *et al.* (2005)
Hyaluronic acid injections relieve knee pain **54**(9): 758–767.

Advice for patients: Information and support for patients

- Arthritis Research Campaign (ARC): ☎ 0870 850 5000
  🖥 www.arc.org.uk
- Arthritis Care: ☎ 0808 800 4050 🖥 www.arthritiscare.org.uk
- The Disabled Living Foundation: ☎ 0870 603 9177
  🖥 www.dlf.org.uk

Rheumatoid arthritis

Rheumatoid arthritis (RA) is the most common disorder of connective tissue affecting ~1% UK population. It is an immunological disease triggered by environmental factors in patients with genetic predisposition. Disease course is variable with exacerbations and remissions.

> ⚠ Refer all suspected cases of rheumatoid arthritis to rheumatology – early treatment with disease-modifying drugs can significantly alter disease progression.

Presentation
- Can present at any age: most common in middle age. $♀:♂ ≈ 3:1$.
- Variable onset: often gradual but may be acute.
- Usually starts with symmetrical small joint involvement i.e. pain, stiffness, swelling and functional loss (especially in the hands) – joint damage and deformity occur later.
- Irreversible damage occurs early if untreated and can → deformity and joint instability.
- Other presentations: monoarthritis; migratory (palindromic) arthritis; PMR-like illness in the elderly; systemic illness of malaise, pain and stiffness.

Symptoms and signs: Predominantly peripheral joints are affected – symmetrical joint pain, effusions, soft tissue swelling, early morning stiffness. Progression to joint destruction and deformity. Tendons may rupture. Specific features – Table 4.9.

Differential diagnosis: Diagnosis may not be easy. *Consider:*
- Psoriatic arthritis
- Nodal OA
- SLE (especially in ♀ <50y.)
- Bilateral carpal tunnel syndrome
- Other connective tissue disorders
- Polymyalgia rheumatica in the elderly.

Investigations
- Check FBC (normochromic, normocytic or hypochromic, microcytic anaemia), ESR and/or CRP (↑). May have ↑platelets, ↓WCC
- Rheumatoid factor and anti-CCP antibodies are +ve in the majority. A minority have a +ve ANA titre
- X-rays: normal, periarticular osteporosis or soft tissue swelling in the early stages; later – loss of joint space, erosions and joint destruction

Management of RA: 📖 p.132

Complications of RA: Physical disability, depression, osteoporosis, ↑ infections, lymphoma, cardiovascular disease, amyloidosis (10%), side effects of treatment.

Further information
Primary Care Rheumatology Society ☎ 01609 774794
🖳 www.pcrsociety.org.uk

Table 4.9 Specific features of rheumatoid arthritis

Hands	• Ulnar deviation of the fingers.
	• 'z' deformity of the thumb.
	• Swan neck (hyperextended PIP and flexed DIP joints) and boutonnière (flexed PIP and extended MCP joints, hyperextended DIP joint) deformities of the fingers (Figure 4.14).
	• ↓ grip strength and ↓ hand function causes disability.
Legs and feet	• Subluxation of the metatarsal heads in feet and claw toes → pain on walking.
	• Baker's cysts (📖 p.106) at the knee may rupture, mimicking DVT.
Spine	Especially cervical spine – causing neck pain, cervical subluxation and atlanto-axial instability leading to a risk of cord compression. X-rays are required prior to general anaesthesia.
Non-articular features	Common. Weight ↓, fever, malaise.
	• *Rheumatoid nodules* (especially extensor surfaces of forearms).
	• *Vasculitis:* digital infarction, skin ulcers, mononeuritis.
	• *Eye:* Sjögren's syndrome, episcleritis, scleritis.
	• *Lungs:* pleural effusions, fibrosing alveolitis, nodules.
	• *Heart:* pericarditis, mitral valve disease, conduction defects.
	• *Skin:* palmar erythema, vasculitis, rashes.
	• *Neurological:* nerve entrapment e.g. carpal tunnel, mononeuritis and peripheral neuropathy.
	• *Felty's syndrome:* combination of RA, splenomegaly and leucopenia. Occurs in patients with long-standing RA. Recurrent infections are common. Hypersplenism → anaemia and thrombocytopenia. Associated with lymphadenopathy, pigmentation and persistent skin ulcers. Splenectomy may improve the neutropenia.

Figure 4.14 Boutonnière and swan neck deformities of the fingers

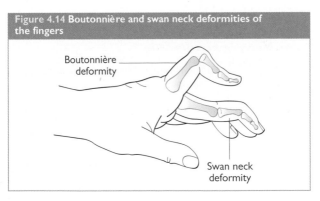

Boutonnière deformity

Swan neck deformity

Management of rheumatoid arthritis

A multidisciplinary team approach is ideal e.g. GP, medical and surgical teams, physiotherapist, podiatrist, OT, nurse specialist and social worker.

General support: Provision of information about the disease, treatments and support available (including equipment and help with everyday activities, self-help and carers, groups, 'blue' disabled parking badges, financial support e.g. DLA, AA – 📖 pp.187–191).

Physical therapy: Exercises, splints, appliances and strapping help to keep joints mobile, ↓ pain and preserve function.

Medication

NSAIDs and simple analgesics: e.g. regular paracetamol. Provide symptomatic relief but do not alter the course of disease. Patients' response to NSAIDs is individual – start with the least gastric toxic e.g. ibuprofen 200–400mg tds and alter as necessary e.g. to diclofenac 50mg tds. A modified release form at night may help early morning symptoms. If the patient has a history of indigestion or gastric problems consider adding gastric protection e.g. misoprostol or a PPI or, if there is no history of ischaemic heart disease or cerebrovascular disease, using a COX2 inhibitor e.g. celecoxib 100mg bd—📖 p.160.

Corticosteroids

- Intra-articular injections of steroids (e.g. Kenalog) can help settle localised flares (e.g. knee or shoulder) and can be used up to 3x/y. in any particular joint.
- Depot IM injections IV or infusions (pulses) can help settle an acute flare but offer short-term benefits with the risk of systemic side effects.
- Daily low-dose oral steroids help symptoms and there is some evidence they can modify disease progression, but concerns about adverse side effects have limited their use.

Disease-modifying drugs (DMARDs)

- Methotrexate
- Gold
- Hydroxychloroquine
- Sulfasalazine
- Azathioprine
- Ciclosporin
- Penicillamine
- Leflunomide
- Cyclophosphamide.
- Cytokine inhibitors (adalimumab, anakinra, etanercept, and infliximab)

Use only under consultant supervision. ↓ disease progression by modifying the immune response and inflammation. Used individually or in combination, they are now started very early in the disease (i.e. first 3–6mo.), hence the need for early referral. DMARDs can take several months to show an effect. Before starting check baseline U&E, Cr, LFTs, FBC and urinalysis. Side effects and monitoring – Table 4.10, 📖 p.136.

Surgery: Aims to relieve pain and improve function. Consideration of the risks, benefits and the most appropriate timing of surgery is vital. *Common procedures:* Joint fusion, replacement and excision; tendon transfer and repair; nerve decompression.

Advice for patients: Information and support for patients

- Arthritis Research Campaign (ARC): ☎ 0870 850 5000
  🖳 www.arc.org.uk
- Arthritis Care: ☎ 0808 800 4050
  🖳 www.arthritiscare.org.uk
- The Disabled Living Foundation: ☎ 0870 603 9177
  🖳 www.dlf.org.uk
- Arthritis Foundation: 🖳 www.arthritis.org

Side effects
- ↑ BP
- Osteoporosis ± fracture
- Proximal muscle wasting
- Euphoria
- Paranoid states or depression, especially if past history
- Peptic ulceration – soluble or EC versions may ↓ risk
- Growth suppression
- Suppression of clinical signs – may allow diseases e.g. septicaemia to reach advanced stage before being recognized
- Spread of infection e.g. chickenpox
- DM and worsening of diabetic control in diabetic patients
- Cushing's syndrome – moon face, striae and acne
- Adrenal atrophy – can persist for years after stopping long-term steroids; illness or surgical emergencies may require steroid supplements
- Na^+ and water retention; K^+ loss

Administration: Often started at high dose to suppress disease process and stepped down with improvement. Use the minimum dose that controls disease as maintenance therapy. Prescribe as a single dose in the morning to ↓ circadian rhythm disturbance. Supply with a 'steroid card' (📖 p.135).

Withdrawal of steroids: Stop abruptly if disease is unlikely to relapse, the patient has received treatment for ≤3wk. and is not included in the patient groups described below.

Withdraw gradually if disease is unlikely to relapse and the patient has:
- recently had repeated steroid courses (particularly if taken for >3wk.)
- taken a short course <1y. after stopping long-term therapy
- other possible causes of adrenal suppression
- received >40mg od of prednisolone (or equivalent)
- been given repeat doses in the evening
- received treatment with steroids for >3wk.

During corticosteroid withdrawal, ↓ dose rapidly to physiological levels (~ prednisolone 7.5mg od) – thereafter ↓ more slowly. Assess the disease during withdrawal to ensure relapse doesn't occur.

Advice for patients: Steroid treatment card

I am a patient on STEROID treatment which must not be stopped suddenly.

- If you have been taking this medicine for more than three weeks, the dose should be reduced gradually when you stop taking steroids unless your doctor says otherwise.
- Read the patient information leaflet given with the medicine.
- Always carry this card with you and show it to anyone who treats you (for example, a doctor, nurse, pharmacist or dentist). For one year after you stop treatment, you must mention that you have taken steroids.
- If you become ill, or if you come into contact with anyone who has an infectious disease, consult your doctor promptly. If you have never had chickenpox, you should avoid close contact with people who have chickenpox or shingles. If you do come into contact with chickenpox, see your doctor urgently.
- Make sure that the information on the card is kept up to date.

Obtaining steroid cards:
- England and Wales: Department of Health ☎ 08701 555 455
- Scotland: Banner Business Supplies ☎ 01506 448 440

Extract reproduced from the Dept. of Health HSC 1998/056: Revised national steroid treatment card, with kind permission of the Crown.

Table 4.10 Specific disease-modifying drugs – side effects and monitoring

⚠ Before starting check baseline U&E, Cr, LFTs, FBC and urinalysis.

Drug	Monitoring	Side effects to monitor
Methotrexate 7.5–30mg weekly Followed the day after by folate 5mg ie weekly as well.	FBC, U&E, Cr and LFTs before starting treatment, weekly for 6wk then every 2–3mo. CXR within 1y. of start of treatment. Check baseline pulmonary function tests in patients with lung disease.	Ask patients to report all symptoms/signs of infection, especially sore throat. Severe respiratory symptoms in the 1st 6mo. – refer to A&E. If MCV >105 fl check B12/folate.

⚠ Advise patients NOT to self-medicate with aspirin or ibuprofen. Avoid alcohol.

Drug	Monitoring	Side effects to monitor
Sulfasalazine 1g bd maintenance	FBC, LFTs + U&E, Cr at 2, 4, 6 & 8wk. then every 4 wk. for 3mo. then 3 monthly. Urgent FBC if intercurrent illness during initiation of treatment.	Rash (1%) Nausea/diarrhoea – often transient. Bone marrow suppression in 1–2% in the first months.If MCV >105fl check B12/folate.
Intramuscular gold (myocristin) 50mg monthly	FBC, urinalysis, ESR, prior to each injection. LFTs, U&E, Cr 3 monthly. CXR within 1y. of start of treatment.	Ask patients to report: All symptoms/signs of infection, especially sore throat Bleeding/bruising Breathlessness/ cough Mouth ulcers/metallic taste in mouth or Rashes
D Penicillamine 375mg–1g/d. maintenance	FBC, urinalysis 2 weekly for 8wk. & 1wk. after any ↑ dosage, then monthly. LFTs and U&E, Cr annually.	Altered taste – can be ignored, rash.
Azathioprine Up to 2.5mg/kg/d. maintenance	FBC weekly for 6wk, 2 and 4 wk. after any dose ↑, then 1x/mo. U&E and LFTs 1x/mo. for 3mo. or until dose stable then 3 monthly.	GI side effects, rash, bone marrow suppression. Avoid live vaccines.

⚠ If allopurinol is co-prescribed, ↓dose to 25% of the original.

Drug	Monitoring	Side effects to monitor
Ciclosporin Up to 3.5mg/kg/d. maintenance	Cr & BP 2 weekly to stable dose then 1x/mo. FBC, U&E, LFTs 1x/mo. until stable for 3mo. then 3 monthly. Lipids 6 monthly.	Rash, gum soreness, hirsitism, ↑ Cr (if ↑ by >30% from baseline, withold and discuss with rheumatologist), ↑BP, renal failure.
Hydroxychloroquine 100–200mg/d. maintenance	Baseline eye check and periodically on advice of local ophthalmologist.	Rash, GI effects, ocular side effects (rare).
Leflunomide 10–20mg/d. maintenance	FBC, LFTs, U&E, BP – 2 weekly for 6mo. then monthly.	Rash, GI, ↑ BP, ↑ ALT

GMS contract			
Records Indicator 8	There is a designated place for the recording of drug allergies and adverse reactions in the notes and these are clearly recorded.	1 point	
Records Indicator 9	For repeat medicines, an indication for the drug can be identified in the records (for drugs added to the repeat prescription with effect from 1 April 2004).	4 points	Minimum standard 80%
Medicines Indicator 12	A medication review is recorded in the notes in the preceding 15 months for all patients being prescribed repeat medicines.	8 points	Minimum standard 80%

Shared – care drug monitoring for penicillamine, auranofin, sulfasalazine, methotrexate & sodium aurothiomalate (myocristin) may be provided by practices as a national enhanced service – 🕮 p.204.

⚠ Results requiring action:

- Total WBC <4.0
- Neutrophils <2
- Platelets <150
- LFTs (ALT/AST) >2x baseline
- Persistent proteinuria (>1+ x2) or haematuria.
Discuss with rheumatologist ± stop medication

Further information

British Society for Rheumatology: *National guidelines for the monitoring of second-line drugs* (2000) 🖳 www.rheumatology.org.uk
BNF: 🖳 www.bnf.org

The spondylarthropathies

A group of inflammatory rheumatic diseases characterised by predominant involvement of axial and peripheral joints and entheses (areas where tendons, ligaments or joint capsules attach to bone). This group includes:

- Ankylosing spondylitis
- Psoriatic arthritis
- Reiter's disease
- Arthritis that accompanies inflammatory bowel disease
- Behçet's syndrome
- Whipple's disease

Sacroiliitis and spondylitis occur with all of them, and they are all associated with the HLA B27 genotype.

Ankylosing spondylitis (AS): Prevalence 1:2000. ♂:♀ ≈ 2½ :1. 95% HLAB27 +ve – prevalence in a population mirrors the frequency of the HLAB27 genotype. Risk of developing AS if HLAB27 +ve ≈ 1:3.

Presentation: Typically presents with morning back pain/stiffness in a young man. Progressive spinal fusion (ankylosis) leads to ↓ spinal movement, spinal kyphosis, sacroiliac (SI) joint fusion, neck hyperextension and neck rotation.

Other features:
- ↓ chest expansion
- Chest pain
- Hip and knee arthritis
- Plantar fasciitis and other enthesopathies
- Iritis
- Crohn's or ulcerative colitis
- Heart disease – carditis, aortic regurgitation, conduction defects
- Osteoporosis
- Psoriaform rashes

Tests:
- *Blood:* FBC – normochromic or microcytic hypochromic anaemia, ↑ ESR (may be normal), RhF usually –ve.
- *X-ray:* Initial signs are widening of the SI joints and marginal sclerosis – later SI joint fusion and a 'bamboo spine' (vertebral squaring and fusion).

Management: *Aims to:*
- ↓ inflammation, pain and stiffness
- Alleviate systemic symptoms e.g. fatigue
- Slow or stop long-term progression of the disease

Primary care management:
- Exercise helps the back pain.
- NSAIDs (e.g. diclofenac 50mg tds) also help pain.
- Refer to rheumatologist early for confirmation of diagnosis, education, disease-modifying drugs (📖 p.136) and advice on appropriate exercise regimes to maintain mobility.

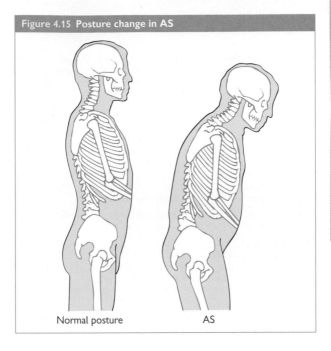

Figure 4.15 Posture change in AS

Normal posture   AS

Advice for patients: Information and support for patients

- National Ankylosing Spondylitis Society (NASS): ☎ 01435 873527
  ▣ www.nass.co.uk
- Arthritis Research Campaign (ARC): ☎ 0870 850 5000
  ▣ www.arc.org.uk

Psoriatic arthritis: Inflammatory arthritis associated with psoriasis (~40% psoriasis patients. ♂ = ♀). 75% patients have a pre-existing history of psoriasis before the arthropathy; in 15% the rash appears simultaneously with the joint symptoms; in 10% the arthritis precedes the skin changes. Presentation is variable. Patterns include:

- **Distal arthritis:** DIP joint swelling of hands/feet, nail dystrophy ± flexion deformity. Sausage-shaped fingers are characteristic of psoriatic arthritis affecting the hand.
- **Rheumatoid-like:** Polyarthropathy similar to rheumatoid arthritis (📖 p.130) but less symmetrical and rheumatoid factor is –ve.
- **Mutilans:** Associated with severe psoriasis. Erosions in small bones of hands/feet ± spine. Bones dissolve → progressive deformity.
- **Ankylosing spondylitis/sacroiliitis:** usually HLA B27 +ve.

Investigations: WBC – usually ↑; ESR/CRP – usually ↑; rheumatoid factor negative; x-ray appearances can be diagnostic.

Management:
- Education; physiotherapy; NSAIDs.
- Refer to rheumatology for confirmation of diagnosis, advice on management and disease-modifying drugs (📖 p.136).
- Medication e.g. methotrexate may improve both skin and musculoskeletal symptoms.

Reactive arthritis: Often asymmetrical aseptic arthritis in ≥1 joint. Occurs 2–6wk. after bacterial infection elsewhere – e.g. gastroenteritis (Salmonella, Campylobacter), GU infection (Chlamydia, Gonorrhoea). ↑ in HLA B27 +ve individuals.

Management:
- NSAIDs, physiotherapy and steroid joint injections.
- Recovery usually occurs within months.
- A minority develop chronic arthritis requiring disease – modifying drugs. Refer to rheumatology.

Reiter syndrome: Polyarthropathy, urethritis, iritis and a psoriaform rash. Affects men with HLA B27 genotype. Commonly follows genitourinary or bowel infection. Joint and eye changes are often severe. Refer for specialist management.

Enteropathic spondylarthropathy: Oligoarticular or polyarticular arthritis linked to inflammatory bowel disease. Presentation is variable and includes: sacroiliitis, plantar fasciitis, inflammatory spinal pains and other enthsitides (insertional ligament/tendon inflammation). Arthritis may evolve and relapse/remit independently of bowel disease.

Management:
- NSAIDs may help joint pain but aggravate bowel disease.
- Refer to rheumatology for confirmation of diagnosis, advice on management and disease-modifying drugs.

Behçet disease: Multi-organ disease. *Cause:* Unknown – thought to be infective. ♂:♀ ≈ 2:1. *Clinical picture (only some features are usually present):* Arthritis; ocular symptoms and signs – pain, ↓ vision, floaters, iritis; scarring painful ulceration of mouth and/or scrotum/labia; colitis; meningoencephalitis.

Management:
- Refer to GUM clinic, ophthalmologist or general physician depending on symptom cluster.
- Treatment is usually with high-dose prednisolone or colchicine.
- Topical steroids may be useful for ulcers.

Advice for patients: Information and support for patients

- Psoriatic Arthropathy Alliance (PAA): ☎ 0870 770 3212
  🖳 www.paalliance.org
- Arthritis Research Campaign (ARC): ☎ 0870 850 5000
  🖳 www.arc.org.uk

Crystal-induced arthritis

Gout: Intermittent attacks of acute joint pain due to deposition of uric acid crystals. *Prevalence:* 3–8/1000. ↑ with age; ♂:♀ ≈ 5:1.

Predisposing factors:
- FH
- Obesity
- Excess alcohol intake
- High-purine diet
- Diuretics
- Acute infection
- Ketosis
- Surgery
- Plaque psoriasis
- Polycythaemia
- Leukaemia
- Cytotoxics
- Renal failure

Presentation of acute gout: Painful swollen joint (big toe, feet and ankles most commonly); red skin which may peel ± fever. Can be polyarticular, especially in elderly ♀. May mimic septic arthritis.

Investigation:
- *Blood:* ↑WCC; ↑ESR; ↑ blood urate (but may be normal).
- *Microscopy of synovial fluid:* not usually required – reveals sodium monourate crystals on polarized light microscopy.
- *X-rays:* not usually required – show soft tissue swelling only, unless severe disease when an erosive pattern is seen.

Management of acute gout:
- Exclude infection.
- Rest and elevate joint – apply ice packs.
- NSAIDs are helpful e.g. diclofenac 75mg bd – caution if GI problems.
- Alternatively, if NSAIDs are contraindicated, try colchicine 500mcg bd increased slowly to qds until pain is relieved or side effects e.g. nausea, vomiting or diarrhoea (max. 6mg – don't repeat in <3d.).
- Steroid joint injection or depomedrone 80–120mg IM are also effective.

Resolves in <2wk. – often after 2–7d. if treated.

Prevention of further attacks:
- ↓ weight
- Avoid alcohol and purine-rich foods (e.g. offal, red meat, yeast extracts, pulses and mussels).
- Avoid thiazide diuretics and aspirin.
- Consider prophylactic medication if recurrent attacks: allopurinol 100–300mg daily – wait until 1mo. after acute attack and co-prescribe colchicine (500mcg bd) or NSAID for first 1–3mo. to try to avoid precipitation of another acute attack. Check serum urate level after 2mo. – aim for low normal range.
- Alternatively or in addition try an uricosuric e.g. probenecid 250–500mcg bd.

Chronic gout: Recurrent attacks, tophi (urate deposits) in pinna, tendons and joints and joint damage. Refer to rheumatology.

Calcium pyrophosphate deposition disease (CPPD): Inflammatory arthritis due to deposition of pyrophosphate crystals. Associated with OA, hyperparathyroidism and haemochromatosis.

Presentation: Attacks are less severe than gout and may be difficult to differentiate from other types of arthritis. Knee, wrist and shoulder are most commonly affected. Acute attacks can be triggered by intercurrent illness and metabolic disturbance.

Investigation: Chondrocalcinosis may be seen on x-ray (calcification of articular cartilage). Presence of joint crystals confirms diagnosis.

Management:
- Treat acute attacks like acute gout.
- A chronic form also occurs – frequently erosive. Refer to rheumatology for confirmation of diagnosis and advice on management and disease-modifying drugs.

GP Notes: Screening and referrals

- Gout may be linked to ↑ risk of hypertension and coronary heart disease – screen patients.
- Refer any patient with gout and kidney stones or recurrent UTI to urology.

Connective tissue diseases

Overlapping group of diseases. The common features of all connective tissue diseases are that they affect many organs, and are associated with fever, malaise, chronic (often relapsing/remitting) course and response to steroids. Often difficult to diagnose – refer if suspected to rheumatology.

Systemic lupus erythematosus (SLE): Rare autoimmune disease. Prevalence: 1 in 3000. ♀:♂ ≈ 9:1. ↑ in Afro-Caribbeans and Asians. Onset 15–40y. Presentation is variable (Table 4.11) – multisystem involvement must be demonstrated to make a diagnosis.

Investigations: Check an autoimmune profile – 95% are ANA (anti-nuclear antibody) +ve. Other immunological abnormalities – ↑ double strained DNA, RhF +ve (40%), ↓ complement (C3, C4). FBC: ↓Hb, ↓WCC, ↑ESR.

Management: Refer to rheumatology for specialist treatment.
- NSAIDs help control symptoms.
- Sunscreens protect skin (can be prescribed as ACBS).
- Steroids are the mainstay of treatment of acute flares (always discuss with a rheumatologist).
- Hydroxychloroquine can improve skin and joint symptoms. Cyclophosphamide, methotrexate and ciclosporin are also used – 📖 p.136.

⚠ Sulfonamides and contraceptive steroids may exacerbate SLE.

Drug-induced lupus: Occurs with:
- Minocycline
- Isoniazid
- Hydralazine
- Procainamide
- Chlorpromazine
- Sulfasalazine
- Losartan *and*
- Anti-convulsants.

Remits slowly when the drug is stopped but may need steroid treatment to settle.

Discoid lupus erythematosus (LE): ≥1 round/oval plaque on the face, scalp or hands. Lesions are well-defined, red, atrophic and scaly ± keratin plugs in dilated follicles. Scarring leaves alopecia on the scalp and may result in hypopigmentation. Internal involvement is not a feature. Investigate as for SLE. Diagnosis is confirmed with lesion biopsy. Treatment is with potent topical steroids and sunscreen. Remission occurs in 40%. 5% develop SLE.

Antiphospholipid syndrome: May occur with SLE or alone. ↑ clotting tendencies. Associated with thrombosis, stroke, migraine, miscarriage, myelitis, myocardial infarction and multi-infarct dementia. If suspected start aspirin 150mg od and refer to rheumatology. May need anticoagulation.

Table 4.11 Presentation of SLE

System	% of patients	Presenting complaints
Joints	95%	• Arthritis • Arthralgia • Myalgia • Tenosynovitis
Skin	80%	• Photosensitivity • Facial 'butterfly' rash • Vasculitic rash • Hair loss • Urticaria • Discoid lesions
Lungs	50%	• Pleurisy • Pneumonitis • Pleural effusion • Fibrosing alveolitis
Kidney	50%	• Proteinuria • ↑BP • Glomerulonephritis • Renal failure
Heart	40%	• Pericarditis • Endocarditis
CNS	15%	• Depression • Psychosis • Infarction • Fits • Cranial nerve lesions
Blood	95%	• Anaemia (very common) • Thrombocytopoenia • Splenomegaly
Fatigue	95%	

Advice for patients: Information and support for patients

- Arthritis Research Campaign (ARC): ☎ 0870 850 5000
  🖳 www.arc.org.uk
- Lupus UK: ☎ 01708 731251 🖳 www.lupusuk.com

Raynaud's syndrome: Intermittent digital ischaemia precipitated by cold or emotion. Fingers ache and change colour: pale → blue → red on rewarming. Usually presents <25y. of age and is idiopathic. *Prevalence:* 3–20%; ♀:♂ >1:1; often abates at the menopause; 5% develop autoimmune rheumatic disease – mainly scleroderma and SLE.

Differential diagnosis:
- Scleroderma ± CREST sydrome
- SLE
- RA
- Drugs e.g. β-blockers
- Trauma
- Smoking
- Arteriosclerosis
- Use of vibrating tools
- Leukaemia
- Polycythaemia rubra vera
- Cold agglutinins
- Thoracic outlet obstruction
- Thrombocytosis
- Monoclonal gammopathies
- Mixed cryoglobulinaemia

Management:
- Advise patients to keep warm – woolly socks/gloves/hat in cold weather, hand warmers, stay inside in the cold.
- Avoid drugs that make the condition worse e.g. β-blockers.
- Stop smoking.
- Nifedipine 10–20mg tds or amlodipine 5mg od help some. Fluoxetine may also be helpful (unlicensed).
- If any associated symptoms or severe symptoms refer for rheumatology advice (urgently for IV vasodilation if critical ischaemia e.g. ulceration or infarcts on fingers).

Polymyositis: Insidious, symmetrical, proximal muscle weakness due to muscle inflammation. Dysphagia, dysphonia and/or respiratory muscle weakness may follow. 25% have a purple rash on cheeks, eyelids and other sun-exposed areas (***dermatomyositis***) ± nail-fold erythema. Creatine kinase levels are ↑. Associated with malignancy in 10% of patients >40y. Refer for confirmation of diagnosis and management advice.

Systemic sclerosis: Rare spectrum of disorders causing fibrosis and skin tightening (scleroderma). Raynaud's is usually present, ± ↑ BP, lung fibrosis, GI symptoms, telangiectasias, polyarthritis and myopathy.

Management: Education and support – treat symptoms e.g. of Raynaud's with nifedipine, amlodipine or angiotensin II receptor blockers.

Prognosis: Variable but early specialist management is vital – refer urgently to rheumatology. CREST syndrome is a variant with better prognosis.

CREST syndrome: Comprises:
- Calcinosis of subcutaneous tissues
- Raynaud's
- Oesophageal motility problems
- Scerodactyly and
- Telagiectasia.

Sjögren's syndrome

Primary Sjögren's syndrome: Under-recognized cause of fatigue and dryness of skin/mucous membranes (may present with dyspareunia). Associated with all autoimmune connective tissue diseases and often presents with nodal OA. Long-term associated with lymphoma. Auto-immune profile is characteristic.

Secondary Sjögren's syndrome: Association of any connective tissue disease (50% have RA) with keratoconjunctivitis sicca (↓ lacrimation → dry eyes) or xerostomia (↓ salivation → dry mouth).

Investigations:
- Collect saliva generated in 10min: <0.5ml/min suggests xerostomia.
- Put a strip of filter paper over the lower lid and measure the distance along the paper that tears are absorbed (Schirmer's test) – <10mm in 5 mins suggests ↓ lacrimation.

Management:
- Refer to rheumatology.
- Provide information and support.
- Use artificial tears for dry eyes.
- Xerostomia may respond to frequent cool drinks, artificial saliva sprays e.g. glandosane or sugar-free gum. Inform the dentist of the diagnosis.
- Skin rashes may respond to anti-malarials.
- Long-term monitoring for mucosal lymphomas is important.

Advice for patients: Information and support for patients

- Raynaud's and Scleroderma Association: ☎ 01270 872776
  🖳 www.raynauds.org.uk
- British Sjögren's Association: ☎ 0121 455 6549
  🖳 www.bssa.uk.net

Polymyalgia rheumatica (PMR) and giant cell arteritis (GCA)

2 clinical syndromes which are part of the same spectrum. *Key features:*
- Both PMR and GCA affect the elderly (rare <50y.)
- 50% of patients with GCA also have PMR
- 15% with PMR also have GCA
- ♀:♂ ≈ 3:1
- Both conditions typically respond rapidly and dramatically to corticosteroids.

Presentation: Diagnosis is clinical.
- *General symptoms:* Both PMR and GCA may present with malaise, anorexia, fever, night sweats, weight loss, depression.
- *PMR – typical symptoms:* proximal symmetrical muscle pain and stiffness worse after rest.
- *GCA – typical symptoms:* unilateral throbbing headache, facial pain, scalp tenderness e.g. on brushing hair and/or jaw claudication. Visual symptoms: amaurosis fugax, diplopia, sudden loss of vision. 30–60% became blind before steroids were used to treat the condition.

Investigation
- *Blood:* ↑ESR (usually >30) ± normocytic anaemia.
- *Temporal artery biopsy:* Refer urgently if GCA is suspected. Biopsy may be -ve even in true cases due to skip lesions. Don't withhold treatment whilst waiting for biopsy – but if the patient has had steroids ≥2wk. +ve biopsy is less likely.
- Exclude other diagnoses depending on symptoms e.g. malignancy, RA, myeloma. For PMR – consider acute neck pain syndromes with referred pain, bilateral shoulder lesions, arthritis, spinal stenosis, acute discitis with referred pain and myositis.

Initial management: Corticosteroids prevent vascular complications, particularly blindness, and rapidly relieve symptoms.
- *GCA:* Prescribe prednisolone 1mg/kg/d. (maximum 60mg od); refer urgently to ophthalmology or rheumatology.
- *PMR:* Prednisolone 15mg od; review after 2–4d. – good response does not confirm diagnosis but suggests treatment should be continued.

Ongoing management
- In all cases, ↓ dose of prednisolone as symptoms allow e.g. by 2.5mg every 4wk. until taking 10mg prednisolone od, then by 1mg/mo. to 5mg od, then more slowly. Check ESR with dose changes.
- Slow steroid reduction regime and recheck ESR if ↑ symptoms.
- At the start of treatment give osteoporosis prophylaxis (📖 p.122) and supply with a steroid card (📖 p.135).
- If concerned about steroid side effects, refer to rheumatology for advice on steroid-sparer drug management.

Prognosis: Most patients require >2y. of treatment. Relapse is common after stopping treatment (50% if stopped after 2y.). If relapse occurs review the diagnosis.

GP Notes: Evaluating PMR Criteria

A person may be regarded as having PMR if ≥3 of the following criteria are present:*
- Bilateral shoulder pain or stiffness
- Onset of illness less than 2 weeks' duration
- Initial ESR greater than 40mm per hour
- Morning stiffness lasting longer than 1 hour
- Age 65 years or more
- Depression and/or weight loss
- Bilateral tenderness in the upper arms

* Reproduced with permission from Bird HA et al. (1979) An evaluation of criteria for polymyalgia rheumatica. Annals of the Rheumatic Diseases **38**(5): 434–9.

Vasculitis

Characterized by inflammation within or around blood vessels ± necrosis. Severity depends on size and site of vessels affected. Systemic vasculitis can be life threatening. *Causes:*
- Idiopathic (50%)
- Connective tissue disease (e.g. RA, SLE)
- Infection (e.g. rheumatic fever, infective endocarditis, Lyme's disease)
- Drugs (e.g. NSAIDs, antibiotics)
- Neoplasia (e.g. lymphoma, leukaemia).

Presentation: Variable – may be confined to the skin or systemic involving joints, kidneys, lungs, gut and nervous system.
- *Skin signs* – palpable purpura (often painful) – usually on lower legs/buttocks.
- *Systemic effects* – fever, night sweats, malaise, weight ↓, myalgia and arthralgia may occur in all types of vasculitis.

Conditions: Table 4.12 – many are rare.

Table 4.12 Vasculitic conditions

Condition	Features	Management
Erythema nodosum	Tender erythematous nodules (1–5cm diameter) on extensor surfaces of limbs (especially shins) ± ankle and wrist arthritis ± fever. ♀:♂≈3:1 *Associations:* Acute sarcoidosis; drugs e.g. oral contraceptives, sulfonamides; infammatory bowel disease – UC, Crohn's; malignancy; TB; Streptococcal infection. 20% of cases are idiopathic with no associations.	Resolves in <8wk., non-scarring. No treatment needed.
Henoch-Schönlein purpura (HSP)	More common in children than adults; ♂ > ♀. Presents with a purpuric rash over buttocks and extensor surfaces. Platelet count is normal. Often follows a respiratory infection. *Other features:* Urticaria, nephritis, joint pains, abdominal pain (may mimic acute abdomen).	Refer to paediatrics for confirmation of diagnosis. Most recover fully without treatment over a few months.

Table 4.12 Contd.

Condition	Features	Management
Polyarteritis nodosa (PAN)	Uncommon in the UK. ♂:♀ ≈ 4:1. Peak incidence in middle age. Multi-system necrotizng vasculitis → aneurysms of medium-sized arteries. Presents with: Tender subcutaneous nodules along the line of arteries, coronary arteritis, ↑BP, mononeuritis multiplex, renal failure and gastrointestinal symptoms. Sometimes associated with hepatitis B.	Refer to rheumatology for angiography to confirm diagnosis, and for advice on management. Treatment is with control of ↑BP, high-dose steroids and cyclophosphamide.
Churg-Strauss syndrome	Associated with asthma. Affects coronary, pulmonary, cerebral and splanchnic circulations. Skin manifestations and mononeuritis can also occur. Diagnosis is based on clinical features and biopsy.	Refer for specialist treatment with high-dose prednisolone ± cyclophosphamide. Avoid leukotriene receptor agonist drugs for control of asthma as may worsen symptoms.
Wegener's granulomatosis	Granulomatous vasculitis. Any organ may be involved and symptoms/signs relate to those affected e.g. mouth ulcers; nasal ulceration with epistaxis/rhinitis; otitis media; cranial nerve lesions; lung symptoms and shadows on CXR; ↑BP; eye signs (50%). Often long prodrome of 'limited Wegener's granulomatosis' – nasal stuffiness, headaches, hearing difficulties and nose bleeds.	Refer to rheumatology/general medicine for investigation. ANCA helps diagnostically and in disease monitoring. Treatment is with high-dose steroids, methotrexate, mofetil and cyclophosphamide.
Kawasaki's disease	Predominantly affects children <5y. Cause unknown. Diagnosis: Diseases with similar presentations have been excluded and ≥5 of: • Fever for ≥5d. • Bilateral conjunctivitis • Polymorphous rash • Changes in lips/mouth – red, dry or cracked lips; strawberry tongue; diffuse redness of mucosa • Changes in extremities – reddening of palms/soles; oedema of hands/feet; peeling of skin of hands, feet and/or groin • Cervical lymphadenopathy >15mm diameter (usually single and painful) ↑ suspicion if poor response to anti-pyretics.	If suspected refer for urgent paediatric assessment. Early treatment (<10d. after onset) with IV immunoglogulin and aspirin ↓ incidence and severity of aneurysm formation as well as giving symptom relief. Complications: Coronary arteritis with formation of aneurysms; accelerated atherosclerosis.

Chronic fatigue syndrome (CFS, ME)

A debilitating and distressing condition. *Prevalence:* 0.2–2.6%; ♀:♂ ≈ 3:2.

Cause: Poorly understood – viral infections (≈10% after EBV), immunization, chemical toxins (e.g. organophosphates, chemotherapy drugs) are all implicated.

Clinical features:* Unexplained fatigue of new/definite onset, not resulting from ongoing exertion, nor alleviated by rest, which results in ↓ activity, and ≥4 of:
- Impaired memory or concentration
- Tender cervical/axillary lymph nodes
- Post-exertional malaise lasting >24h.; typically delayed – usually starting 1–2d. after a period of ↑ physical/mental activity – and may last weeks.
- Headaches of new type pattern or severity
- Multi-joint pain without swelling
- Sore throat
- Unrefreshing sleep
- Muscle pain

Additional symptoms must not have pre-dated fatigue.

🕐 Diagnostic criteria require the fatigue to have been present for ≥6mo.* but most patients present to general practice long before that.

Other common symptoms/associations
- Postural dizziness
- Vertigo
- Altered temperature sensation
- Paraesthesiae
- Sensitivity to light or sound
- Palpitations
- IBS
- Food intolerance
- Fibromyalgia
- Feelings of dyspnoea
- Mood swings
- Panic attacks
- Depression (60% have no prior psychiatric diagnosis)

Intercurrent infection, immunization, drugs, caffeine, alcohol and stress may → setbacks.

Management
- Support and reassurance – explanation, information ± self-help groups.
- Avoid factors which worsen symptoms e.g. caffeine, alcohol.
- Graded exercise is helpful^C.
- Treat symptoms e.g. TCA (e.g. amitriptyline 10–50mg nocte – unlicensed) to help sleep, relieve headache or neuropathic pain; SSRI for depression.
- Referral for specialist care e.g. CBT (↓ 2° distress and optimizes rehabilitation), specialist chronic fatigue clinic.

* Fukuda K et al. (1994) The chronic fatigue syndrome: a comprehensive approach to its definition and study. *Annals of Internal Medicine* **121**: 953–9.

Prognosis: Variable. Children tend to recover though it may take years. 55% of adults presenting with tiredness have symptoms lasting >6mo. Risk ↑ 3x if there is a history of anxiety or depression. Short duration of fatigue with no anxiety/depression improves prognosis. Only 6% of adults with CFS attending specialist clinics return to pre-morbid functioning.

Further information

Royal Australian College of Physicians: Chronic Fatigue Syndrome ⊞ www.mja.com.au/public/guides/cfs/cfs1.html
King's College ⊞ www.kcl.ac.uk/cfs

GP Notes: Diagnosing CFS

- Making the diagnosis of chronic fatigue syndrome is seen by patients as the most helpful thing a GP can do.
- Uncomplicated depression does not exclude a diagnosis of CFS – the 2 frequently co-exist.
- Exclusion criteria for diagnosis include:
  - Active disease likely to cause fatigue
  - Psychotic disorders – including schizophrenia and bipolar disorder
  - Anorexia and bulimia
  - Dementia
  - Substance abuse – alcohol and drugs *and*
  - Severe obesity

Advice for patients: Information and support for patients

- ME Association: ☎ 0871 222 7824
  ⊞ www.meassociation.org.uk
- Action for ME: ☎ 01749 670799 ⊞ www.afme.org.uk
- Royal College of Psychiatrists–patient information sheets:
  ⊞ www.rcpsych.ac.uk

Fibromyalgia

Painful, non-articular condition of unknown cause, predominantly involving muscles. Fibromyalgia is common and often results in significant disability and handicap with inability to cope with a job or household activities. Peak age 40–50y. – 90% female.

Clinical picture
- Pain: usually axial and diffuse but may be felt all over.
- Pain is worsened by stress, cold and activity and associated with generalized morning stiffness.
- Paraesthesiae or dysaesthesiae of hands and feet are common.
- Analgesics, NSAIDs and local physical treatments are ineffective and may worsen symptoms.
- Sleep patterns are poor: patients tend to wake exhausted and complain of poor concentration.
- Anxiety and depression scores are high.
- Associated symptoms: unexplained headache, urinary frequency and abdominal symptoms are common.
- Clinical findings are unremarkable.

Investigation: Exclude other causes of pain and fatigue (e.g. hypothyroidism, SLE, Sjögren's psoriatic arthritis, inflammatory myopathy, hyperparathyroidism, osteomalacia) – check FBC, ESR, TFTs, U&E, Ca^{2+}, CK, PO_4, ANA, Rh.F and immunoglobulins.

Diagnostic criteria
- History of widespread pain (defined as pain on both left and right sides, above and below the waist, together with axial skeletal pain e.g. neck or back pain), *in combination with*
- Pain in ≥11 out of 18 tender points sites (Figure 4.16) on digital palpation.

Management: A multidisciplinary approach is helpful – usually accessed through a rheumatology or pain clinic.
- Be supportive: reassurance that there is no serious pathology, explanation and information are vital.
- Low-dose amitriptyline 25–75mg nocte may help with sleep and pain.
- SSRI e.g. sertraline 25–50mg od may help anxiety, depression and sleep – stop if no improvement after a month's trial.
- Graded exercise regimes can improve pain, lethargy, mood and general malaise.
- Counselling and learning of coping strategies can be beneficial as can cognitive behavioural therapy if available locally.
- Some patients benefit from injection of hypalgesic trigger points with steroid or acupuncture to trigger points.

Figure 4.16 Tender points sites for diagnosis of fibromyalgia

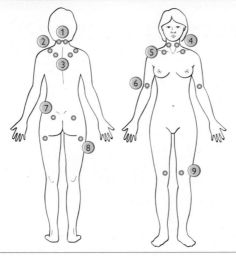

1. Insertion of nuchal muscles into the occiput
2. Upper border of trapezius midportion
3. Muscle attachments to upper medial border of scapula
4. Anterior aspects of the C5, C7 intertransverse spaces
5. 2nd rib space ~3cm lateral to the sternal border
6. Muscle attachments to the lateral epicondyle at the elbow
7. Upper outer quadrant of gluteal muscles
8. Muscle attachments just posterior to the greater trochanter
9. Medial fat pad of the knee just proximal to the joint line

Advice for patients: Information and support for patients

- Arthritis Research Campaign (ARC): ☎ 0870 850 5000
  🖳 www.arc.org.uk
- Fibromyalgia Association UK: ☎ 0870 220 1232
  🖳 www.fibromyalgia-associationuk.org
- STIFF (UK): ☎ 01782 562 366 🖳 www.stiffuk.org

Miscellaneous conditions

Neuropathic arthritis: Charcot's disease is a rapidly progressive degeneration in a joint which lacks position sense and protective pain sensation. Upper limb disease is usually associated with syringomyelia. Lower limb disease is usually associated with diabetic neuropathy or cauda equine lesions. The joint may be very deformed but is usually painless. Treat the underlying condition (e.g. diabetes) accordingly. The joint cannot recover but refer to orthopaedics for advice on stabilization.

Haemophiliac arthropathy: Both factor VIII and factor IX haemophilia can cause progressive joint destruction through repeated bleeding into the joints. Risk of bleed is predicted by factor levels – spontaneous bleeds occur if the patient has levels <5% normal. All haemophiliacs need long-term follow-up via a specialist haemophilia centre. Treatment aims to prevent bleeding through prophylaxis (e.g. with tranexamic acid, desmopressin or prophylactic factor VIII or IX) and to minimize the effect of bleeds by on-demand administration of the missing clotting factors as soon as bleeding starts.

Over-training syndrome: Poor performance, fatigue, heavy muscles and depression due to excessive sports training or competing without sufficient rest. Usually diagnosed from history. Exclude other causes of fatigue (📖 p.152). *Management:* Rest, reassurance and alteration of training programme.

Tietze syndrome: Idiopathic costochondritis. Pain is enhanced by motion, coughing or sneezing. The 2nd rib is most commonly affected. Examination: Marked localized tenderness. Differential diagnosis: Muscular sprain; rarely inflammatory chest wall enthesitis/osteitis 2° sponylarthopathy.

Management: Explanation and reassurance that nothing serious is happening; simple OTC analgesia e.g. ibuprofen 400mg tds. If pain persists local steroid or marcaine injections can be helpful. If not settling consider referral to rheumatology.

Musculoskeletal sarcoid: Arthralgia typically of the ankles associated with changes of acute sarcoid. Chronic sarcoid can be associated with erosive arthritis and osteitis/periostitis pains. Erosive arthritis is treated effectively with methotrexate. Refer to rheumatology.

Reflex sympathetic dystrophy (algodystrophy, complex regional pain disorder): Pain ± vasomotor changes in a limb → loss of function and stiffness. Most common in the hand and wrist. Usually follows trauma (but the trauma may be trivial and signs may appear weeks or months later). *Signs:* Pain at rest exacerbated by movement and light touch, swelling, discoloration, temperature changes, abnormal sensitivity, sweating, ↑ hair/nail growth and stiffness. X-ray may show osteopoenia.

Management: Physiotherapy (improves prognosis if started early), analgesia (NSAIDs). Refer to pain clinic and/or rheumatology for IV bisphosphonates (responds well if treated early) and 'mirror' therapy.

Ekbom syndrome (restless legs syndrome): The patient (who is usually in bed) is seized by an irresistible desire to move their legs in a repetitive way accompanied by an unpleasant sensation deep in the legs. Sleep disturbance is common, as is +ve FH (>90%). *Cause:* unknown.

Management:

- Exclude drug causes – common culprits: β-blockers, H_2 antagonists, neuroleptics, lithium, tricyclic antidepressants, anticonvulsants.
- Exclude peripheral neuropathy or ischaemic rest pain.
- Iron deficiency (with or without anaemia) is associated in 1:3 sufferers, so check FBC and serum ferritin.
- Can be secondary to renal disease, DM or hypothyroidism, so check U&E, Cr, fasting blood glucose and TFTs.
- Try non-drug measures first – simple reassurance and information, walking/stretching, warmth (heat pads or warm bath), relaxation exercises, massage.
- Codeine (30–60mg tds/qds), carbamazepine (100mg bd) and clonazepam (1–4mg nocte) may be helpful. Other drugs which have been used include gabapentin and zopiclone. ❶ No drugs are licensed in the UK.
- Refer to neurology or general medicine if severe symptoms or diagnosis is in doubt.

GP Notes: Questions to screen for restless legs

1. Do you or have you ever had an urge to move your legs, usually accompanied or caused by uncomfortable and unpleasant sensations in your legs?
2. Does this urge to move or do these unpleasant sensations begin or worsen during periods of rest or inactivity such as lying down or sitting?
3. Is this urge to move or are these unpleasant sensations partially or totally relieved by movement (e.g. walking or stretching) for at least as long as that activity lasts?
4. Is this urge to move or are these unpleasant sensations worse during the evening or night than they are during the day or do they only occur during the evening or at night?

If the answer to all these questions is 'Yes', a diagnosis of restless legs syndrome is likely.

Advice for patients: Information and support for patients

- Restless Leg Syndrome Foundation: ▯ www.rls.org
- Ekbom Support Group: ▯ www.ekbom.org.uk

Chronic pain control

Pain is always subjective so take it at face value in *all* patients. 7% of adults in the UK have chronic pain. Chronic pain is usually multifactorial.

Assessment: 📖 p.2

Goals of pain management

- Set realistic targets.
- Abolition of pain may be impossible – 70% have pain despite analgesia.
- If analgesia is not helping – stop it.
- The aim is often rehabilitation with ↓ in distress/disability.

Strategies for pain management: A multidisciplinary approach is essential. *Consider:*

- *Prevention:* e.g. wrist splints for carpal tunnel syndrome; analgesia prior to minor surgery.
- *Removal of cause:* Treat medical causes of pain e.g. infection, ↓ blood sugar (diabetic neuropathy). Refer surgical causes for surgery if surgery appropriate e.g. OA – joint replacement.
- *Pain-relieving drugs:* Start with a single drug at low dose and step up dose or add another drug as needed – Figure 4.17. Especially in situations of acute pain, step down if pain diminishes.
- *Physical therapies:* Acupuncture, physiotherapy or TENS.
- *Nerve blocks:* Consider referral for epidural (low back pain), local nerve block or sympathectomy (e.g. vascular rest pain).
- *Modification of emotional response:* Psychotropic drugs e.g. anxiolytics, antidepressants.
- *Modification of behavioural response:* e.g. back pain – consider referral to rehabilitation scheme.

Neuropathic pain: Sharp or burning pain. Typically does not respond well to ordinary analgesia. Tends to be associated with numbness around the area of pain and may be less troublesome when the patient is distracted.

- Try antidepressants (e.g. amitriptyline – 10–25mg nocte increasing as needed every 2wk. to 75–150mg)treatment should start to have an effect within 2wk.
- If unsuccessful consider anticonvulsants (e.g. gabapentin, car-bamazepine, phenytoin, sodium valproate or clonazepam) at standard anticonvulsant dosages.
- Local treatments are sometimes helpful e.g. capsaicin cream.

🚫 If history of penetrating trauma, consider a neuroma (+ve Tinel's test over the trigger point).

Referral: If unable to remove cause and unable to achieve adequate pain relief, consider referral to a specialist pain control clinic.

Further information

OUP: Moore *et al. Bandolier's little book of pain* (2003) ISBN: 0192632477
The Oxford Pain Internet Site:
🖥 www.jr2.ox.ac.uk/bandolier/booth/painpag

Figure 4.17 WHO analgesics ladder

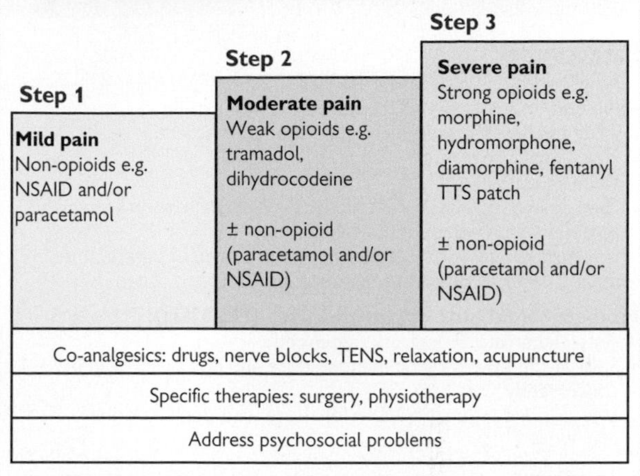

Step 1

Mild pain
Non-opioids e.g.
NSAID and/or
paracetamol

Step 2

Moderate pain
Weak opioids e.g.
tramadol,
dihydrocodeine

± non-opioid
(paracetamol and/or
NSAID)

Step 3

Severe pain
Strong opioids e.g.
morphine,
hydromorphone,
diamorphine, fentanyl
TTS patch

± non-opioid
(paracetamol and/or
NSAID)

Co-analgesics: drugs, nerve blocks, TENS, relaxation, acupuncture

Specific therapies: surgery, physiotherapy

Address psychosocial problems

GP Notes:

⚠ Be aware of 2° gain from pain if symptoms seem out of proportion (outstanding compensation claims are a significant factor in success of pain management).

Pain-relieving drugs

Paracetamol
- As effective a painkiller as ibuprofen.
- No anti-inflammatory effect but potent anti-pyretic.
- Drug of choice in OA where inflammation is absent.
- Side effects are rare.
- Dose 1g qds.
- Overdose (>4g/24h.) can be fatal, causing hepatic damage, sometimes not apparent for 4–6d.
- Inadvertant overdosage is easy due to presence of paracetamol in most OTC cold preparations – refer to A&E.

Non-steroidal anti-inflammatories (NSAIDs): Table 4.13
- Anti-inflammatory, analgesic, antipyretic.
- Start at the lowest recommended dose and don't use >1 NSAID concurrently.
- 60% respond to any NSAID – for those who don't, another may work.

Side effects:
GI side effects: Common (50%) including GI bleeds (¼ GI bleeds in UK). ↑ with age. Risks are dose related and vary between drugs.
- For the elderly, those on steroids or with past history of GI ulceration or indigestion, protect the stomach with misoprostol or PPI.
- Selective inhibitors of cyclo-oxygenase-2 (COX2) are equally effective but should not be given to any patient with pre-existing or high risk of cardio- or cerebrovascular disease.

Other side effects:
- Hypersensitivity reactions 5–10% asthmatics develop bronchospasm
- Fluid retention – relative contraindication in patients with ↑BP/cardiac failure
- Renal failure – rare – commoner in patients with pre-existing renal disease
- Hepatic impairment – particularly diclofenac.

🛈 COX2 inhibitors have NO effect on platelet aggregation; they have no benefit if used in patients on continuous low-dose aspirin; and, there is no evidence combining a COX2 inhibitor with PPI/misoprostol gives extra stomach protection.

Topical NSAIDs: Of proven benefit for acute and chronic conditions and can be as effective as oral preparations. They have lower incidence of GI and other side effects though these still occur.

Opioids: Chronic pain may not respond to an opiate. Give for a 2wk. trial and only continue if of proven benefit. Worries of tolerance/addiction are unfounded for patients with true opioid-sensitive pain. Start at low dose and slowly titrate dose up according to response. Consider providing prophylactic laxatives to prevent constipation.

Combination analgesics

- Combining 2 analgesics with different mechanisms of action enables better pain control than using either drug alone at that dose.
- Combinations have ↓ dose-related side effects but the range of side effects is ↑ (additive effects of 2 drugs).
- In general practice the commonest combinations are aspirin or paracetamol with a mild opiate (e.g. co-codamol). These combinations are no more effective than paracetamol alone but have more side effects and are more dangerous in overdose.
- Combinations using full-dose opiate (e.g. solpadol) are more effective than paracetamol alone but it is cheaper and more flexible if constituents are prescribed separately.

Table 4.13 Commonly used NSAIDs

Drug	Dosage	Features
Ibuprofen	1.2–1.8g/d. in 3–4 divided doses	Fewer side effects than other NSAIDs. Anti-inflammatory properties are weaker. Don't use if inflammation is prominent e.g. gout.
Naproxen	0.5–1g/d. in 1–2 divided doses	Good efficacy with a low incidence of side effects.
Diclofenac	75–150mg/d. in 1–2 divided doses	
Meloxicam	7.5–15mg od	Selective COX2 inhibitors. As effective as non-selective NSAIDs and share side effects but risk of serious upper GI events is lower. Only use it at low risk of cerebro- or cardiovascular disease and high risk of GI side effects[N].
Celecoxib	200mg od or bd	

GP Notes: Use of NSAIDs

- All NSAIDs are associated with GI toxicity – risk is ↑ in the elderly.
- Use lower-risk NSAIDs e.g. ibuprofen as first-line treatment.
- Start at the lowest recommended dose.
- Don't use >1 oral NSAID at a time.
- Remember *all* NSAIDs are contraindicated in patients with active peptic ulceration. Non-selective NSAIDs are contraindicated in patients with a history of peptic ulceration.

❶ Combination of a NSAID and low-dose aspirin may ↑ risk of GI side effects: only use this combination if absolutely necessary and if the patient is monitored closely.

COX2 inhibitors: Due to concerns about cardiovascular safety, *only* use COX2 inhibitors in preference to standard NSAIDs when specifically indicated (i.e. for patients at high risk of developing gastroduodenal ulcer, perforation, or bleeding) and after an assessment of cardiovascular risk. Switch patients receiving a COX2 inhibitor who have ischaemic heart disease or cerebrovascular disease to alternative treatment.

Chronic disease management

The predominant disease pattern in the developed world is one of chronic or long-term illness. In the UK, 17.5 million adults are currently living with a chronic disease. Patient with all types of arthritis are included in this group. Although details of chronic illness management depend on the illness, people with chronic diseases of all types have much in common with each other. *They all:*

- Have similar concerns and problems
- Must deal not only with their disease(s) but also the impact it has on their lives and emotions.

Common elements of effective chronic illness management

Involvement of the whole family: Chronic diseases do not only affect the patient but everyone in a family.

Collaboration between service providers and patients/carers:
- Negotiate and agree a definition of the problem.
- Agree targets and goals for management.
- Develop an individualized self-management plan.

Personalized written care plan: Take into account patient/carers' views and experience and the current evidence base.

Tailored education in self-management: A patient with arthritis spends ~3h./y. with a health professional – the other 8757 h. they manage their own condition. Helping patients with chronic disease understand and take responsibility for their condition is imperative. User-led (i.e. led by someone who suffers from the condition) self-management education programmes are most effective and are becoming increasingly available.

Planned follow-up: Pro-active follow-up according to the care plan – use of disease registers and call–recall systems are important.

Monitoring of outcome and adherence to treatment:
- Use of disease and treatment markers
- Monitoring of compliance e.g. checking prescription frequency
- Medicine management programmes

Tools and protocols for stepped care:
- Provide a framework for using limited resources to greatest effect.
- Step professional care in intensity.
- Start with limited professional input and systematic monitoring.
- Augment care for patients who do not achieve an acceptable outcome.
- Initial and subsequent treatments are selected according to evidence-based guidelines in light of a patient's progress.

Targeted use of specialist services: For those patients who cannot be managed in primary care alone.

Monitoring of process: Continually monitor management of patients with chronic disease through clinical governance mechanisms. Ensure changes are made promptly to optimize care.

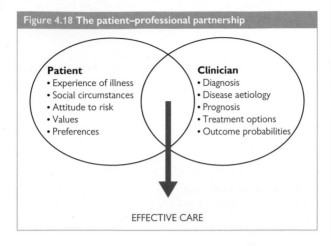

Figure 4.18 The patient–professional partnership

Patient
- Experience of illness
- Social circumstances
- Attitude to risk
- Values
- Preferences

Clinician
- Diagnosis
- Disease aetiology
- Prognosis
- Treatment options
- Outcome probabilities

EFFECTIVE CARE

GP Notes: Common patient concerns may include

- Finding and using health services
- Finding and using other community resources
- Knowing how to recognize and respond to changes in a chronic disease
- Dealing with problems and emergencies
- Making decisions about when to seek medical help
- Using medicines and treatments effectively
- Knowing how to manage stress and depression that accompany a chronic illness
- Coping with fatigue, pain and sleep problems
- Getting enough exercise
- Maintaining good nutrition
- Working with your doctor(s) and other care providers
- Talking about your illness with family and friends
- Managing work, family and social activities

Expert patient schemes:
Aim to train people with long-term chronic conditions to 'self-manage' their conditions more objectively on a day-to-day basis. Further information is available from 🖳 www.expertpatients.nhs.uk

Further information

Von Korff et al. (2002) Organising care for chronic illness. BMJ **325**: 92–4.

Rehabilitation

'Use strengthens, disuse debilitates'
Hippocrates (460–357 BC)

13–14% of the population have some disability. This is increasing as populations age and people survive longer with disability. Most patients are best managed by a multidisciplinary team in their home environment (if practicable) with a problem-oriented approach. Good interdisciplinary communication and co-ordination is essential and many patients benefit from specialist rehabilitation services. Psychological and sociocultural aspects are as important as medical aspects.

Principles of rehabilitation

- *Use of assessments/measures:* Central to management of any disability. Use validated measures accepted by all team members. Reassess regularly.
- *Teamwork:* Good outcomes are associated with clinicians working as a team towards a common goal with patients and their families (or carers) included as team members.
- *Goal setting:* Goals must be meaningful, challenging but achievable. Use short- and long-term goals. Involve the patient ± carer(s). Regularly renew, review and adapt.
- *Underlying approach to therapy:* All approaches focus on modification of impairment and improvement in function within everyday activities. Patients derive benefit from therapy focused on the management of disability.
- *Intensity/duration of therapy:* How much therapy is needed? Is there a minimum threshold below which there is no benefit at all? Studies on well-organized services show it is rare for patients to receive >2h. therapy/d. No one knows what is ideal.

Role of the GP

- The GP of any patient receiving rehabilitation in the community is a team member and may be the key worker who co-ordinates care.
- Maintain an open door policy and encourage patients and carers to seek help for problems early.
- Try to become familiar with a patient's disease, even if it is rare. It is impossible to plan care without knowledge of course and prognosis, and an easy way to lose a patient's confidence if you appear ignorant of their condition.
- If progress is slower than expected, or stalls, consider other medical problems (e.g. anaemia, hypothyroidism, dementia), a neurological event, depression and communication problems (e.g. poor vision/hearing).
- Information alone can improve outcome.

Care of informal carers: 📖 p.166

Benefits: 📖 pp.179–193

GP Notes: Checklist of areas to cover

- Can physical symptoms be improved?
- Can the psychological symptoms be improved (including self-esteem)?
- Can functioning within the home be improved? (aids and
- adaptations within the home, extra help)
- Can functioning in the community be improved? (mobility outside the home, work, social activities)
- Can the patient's or carer's financial state be improved? (benefits)
- Does the carer need more support? (voluntary and self-help organizations, social services)

Advice for patients: Information and support for patients and carers

- Support organisations for the patient's condition (e.g. Arthritis Foundation) – 📖 p.212
- Department of Work and Pensions: 🖥 www.dwp.gov.uk
  ☎ *Benefits Enquiry Line* – 0800 882200; 0800 243355 (minicom facility); 0800 441144 (for help with form completion)
- Citizens' Advice Bureau: 🖥 www.adviceguide.org.uk
- Age Concern: ☎ 0800 009966 🖥 www.ageconcern.org.uk
- Help the Aged: ☎ 0800 800 65 65
  🖥 www.helptheaged.org.uk
- Disabled Living Foundation – advice about equipment and appliances: ☎ 0845 130 9177 🖥 www.dlf.org.uk
- Royal Association for Disability and Rehabilitation (RADAR):
  ☎ 020 7250 3222 🖥 www.radar.org.uk
- Disablement Information and Advice Line (DIAL): ☎ 01302 310123

Care of informal carers

In the UK there are 6 million informal carers who are vitally important to the well-being of disabled people in the community. Most are relatives or friends of the person being cared for. Many are elderly with health problems themselves. There is good evidence their health suffers as a result of caring – 52% report treatment for a stress-related illness since becoming a carer and 51% report being physically injured as a result of caring.

GPs and their primary care teams are often the 1st point of access for any help needed and 88% of carers have seen their GP in the past 12 mo. Carers see the GP as the professional most able to improve their lives but few GPs have had any training about their problems and 71% carers believe their GPs are unaware of their needs.

Physical help: Record whether a patient is a carer in their notes.
- *Practical advice on nursing skills:* Ask DNs to review problems.
- *Advice on management:* Specialist nurses (e.g. CPNs etc.) provide special expertise.
- *Additional help:* Social services can provide home care. Voluntary organisations provide sitting services e.g. Crossroads schemes. Every carer has a right to ask for a full assessment of their needs by the social services.
- *Home modification:* Local authorities can arrange modifications. DNs have access to equipment needed for nursing. The Red Cross loans commodes, wheelchairs etc.
- *Respite:* Hospitals, charity organisations and local authorities provide day care (to give regular breaks each week) and respite care (for a week or more at a time).

Emotional support
- *Self-help carers groups:* Opportunity to share experiences with people in similar situations.
- *Always ask the carer how they are when visiting* – even if they are not your patient themselves.
- *If the patient and/or carer have a religion, the clergy will often provide ongoing support.*
- *Maintain good lines of communication.* Treat the carer as a team member. Make sure you inform both carer and patient fully. Make appointments for review. Don't be short with a carer, patronising or impossible to contact.

Financial support: Many patients who have carers are entitled to Attendance Allowance or Disability Living Allowance (📖 p.188). If the patient is not expected to live >6mo. they are entitled to claim under Special Rules. This benefit is *not* means tested. Other benefits:
- *Low income:* 📖 pp.184–186
- *Given up work to look after the patient:* May be eligible for carers allowance – 📖 p.189.
- *Substantial modification to home:* Council tax may be payable at lower rate (consult local council).

GMS contract

Management Indicator 9	The practice has a protocol for the identification of carers and a mechanism for the referral of carers for social services assessment	3 points

Advice for patients: Support organizations for carers

- Carers UK: ☎ 020 7490 8818 🖳 www.carersonline.org.uk
- Princess Royal Trust for Carers: ☎ 020 7480 7788
  🖳 www.carers.org
- Support organizations for the patient's condition (e.g. Arthritis Foundation) – 📖 p.212
- Department of Work and Pensions: 🖳 www.dwp.gov.uk
  ☎ Benefits Enquiry Line – 0800 882200; 0800 243355 (minicom facility); 0800 441144 (for help with form completion)
- Citizens' Advice Bureau: 🖳 www.adviceguide.org.uk
- Age Concern: ☎ 0800 009966 🖳 www.ageconcern.org.uk
- Help the Aged: ☎ 0800 800 65 65 🖳 www.helptheaged.org.uk
- Counsel and Care: ☎ 0845 300 7585
  🖳 www.counselandcare.org.uk

GP Notes: Carer skills

A carer skills course is being developed for the expert patient programme. Further information is available at 🖳 www.expertpatients.nhs.uk

Chapter 5

Joint injection techniques

'A minor operation: one performed on someone else'
Unaccredited Penguin Dictionary of
Humorous Quotations (2001)

Providing joint and soft tissue injections

Steroids can have a potent local anti-inflammatory effect and dramatically improve certain musculoskeletal problems. Most joint injections are straightforward and can be undertaken within a general practice setting.

Preparation for the procedure

- Take a history, make a careful examination and have a clear diagnosis before considering injecting steroids.
- Gather the needles, syringes, a sterile container (for sending aspirated fluid to the laboratory), steroid, local anaesthetic, skin preparation fluid (e.g. chlorhexidine), cotton wool and elastoplast beforehand.
- The injected joint should be rested for 2–3d. afterwards if possible – certainly avoid heavy activity. Make sure the patient is comfortable, has given informed consent and knows what to expect.

Consent: Patient consent for the procedure must be sought and recorded in the notes. This involves giving enough information about the procedure and other possible treatment options to allow the patient to make an informed decision about whether to proceed; the patient and consenting doctor should then both sign the consent form and the form should be filed in the patient's medical records.

 Part of the specification for a directed enhanced service for minor surgery includes the use of a standard NHS consent form available via the Department of Health website (🖥 www.dh.gov.uk).

Steroid preparations: (↑ order of potency) hydrocortisone acetate, methylprednisolone acetate, triamcinolone hexacetonide.

Local anaesthetic (LA): e.g. lidocaine 1% can be mixed with the steroid for some injections – LA effect occurs immediately and lasts 2–4h. The patient may then experience some return of symptoms (pain) before the steroid takes effect – warn the patient.

Follow-up

- Some injections are painful at administration – this is normal for tennis elbow and plantar faciitis.
- Severe or increasing pain ~48h. after injection may indicate sepsis – advise the patient to return urgently if this occurs.
- If steroid is injected close to the skin surface (as in tennis elbow), skin dimpling and pigment loss can occur – warn the patient.

⚠ Never attempt a procedure if you are unsure about it – know the boundaries of your experience and abilities.

GMS contract

Minor surgery can be provided as an additional service or directed enhanced service (□ p.202).

| *Management Indicator 4* | The arrangements for instrument sterilization comply with national guidelines as applicable to primary care | 1 point |

GP Notes: General rules

- Always use aseptic technique.
- Do not inject if there is local sepsis (e.g. cellulitis) or any possibility of joint infection.
- Never inject into the substance of a tendon – this may cause rupture (in tenosynovitis steroid is injected into the tendon sheath).
- Injections should not require pressure on the syringe plunger – if so the needle is probably not correctly located (tennis elbow is an exception).
- Undertake as few injections as possible to settle the problem – often 1 is sufficient. If no improvement after 2–3 then reconsider the diagnosis.
- Do no more than 3–4 injections/patient/appointment and no more than 3–4 in any single joint/year – more than this ↑ risk of systemic absorption and joint damage.

Advice for patients: Information and support for patients

Arthritis Research Campaign (ARC) – patient information leaflet 'Local Steroid Injections': ☎ 0870 850 5000 🖳 www.arc.org.uk

Further information

Radcliffe Publishing: Silver T. *Joint and soft tissue injection: injecting with confidence* (2001) ISBN 1 85775 143 4

Most hospital rheumatology departments have a joint injection clinic and are happy to allow GPs to watch to gain experience.

Lower limb injections

The knee: Joint effusions are common (e.g. trauma, ligament strains, OA, RA, gout). Aspiration of fluid can:
- Help make a diagnosis e.g. gout
- Be a therapeutic procedure – draining a tense effusion can relieve pain
- Precede administration of steroids e.g. RA flare.

Aspirated fluid should be clear or slightly yellow and not purulent. If aspirating an effusion, send the fluid for analysis.

⚠ Any sign of infection within the joint prohibits steroid use.

Technique for aspiration and joint injection
- Lie the patient on couch with knee slightly bent – place a pillow under the knee as this relaxes the muscles.
- Palpate the joint space under the lateral or medial edge of the patella and inject/aspirate just below the superior border of the patella with the needle horizontal – Figure 5.1.
- Use a green (21 gauge) needle.
- If aspirating and then injecting steroids maintain the needle in position and swap the syringe.
- Normal doses of steroid are triamcinolone 20mg or methylprednisolone 40mg.
- In prepatella bursitis, aspiration and injection of hydrocortisone 25mg into the bursa can help settle inflammation.

Plantar fasciitis: Painful area in the middle of the heel pad can be helped by steroid injection into the most tender spot – it hurts so advise analgesia. Mixing lidocaine 1% with the steroid (e.g. triamcinolone 10–20mg) can help.

Technique: Two methods are commonly used (Figure 5.2):
- Injection through the tough skin of the sole of the foot (more accurate) or
- Lateral approach (less painful).

Rest the foot for several days and use an in-shoe heel pad. Rupture of the plantar fascia is a rare complication.

Figure 5.1 Knee joint injection

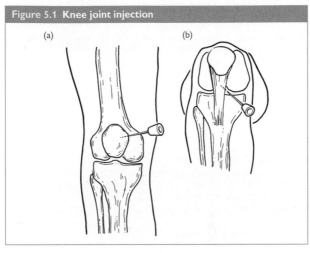

Reproduced with kind permission of the British Journal of Hospital Medicine.

Figure 5.2 Injection of plantar fasciitis

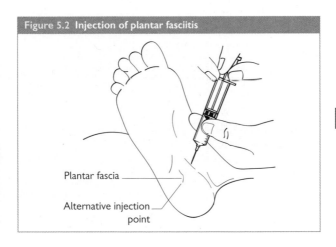

Plantar fascia

Alternative injection point

Upper limb injections

Tenosynovitis: Causes pain and stiffness in the line of the tendon, and crepitus over the affected tendon. The most common site is the base of the thumb (DeQuervain's tenosynovitis).

Injecting steroid and local anaesthetic (e.g. hydrocortisone 25mg and 1ml 1% lignocaine) into the space between the tendon and the sheath can help.

Technique
- Insert the needle along the line of the tendon just distal to the point of maximum tenderness.
- Advance the needle proximally into the tendon (felt as a resistance) and then slowly withdraw until the resistance disappears. The tip of the needle is now in the tendon sheath.
- It is now safe to inject – the tendon sheath may swell.
- Advise the patient to rest the affected area for several days and avoid the precipitating activity.

Carpal tunnel syndrome: Can be relieved by steroid injection.

Technique
- Sit the patient with hand resting on a firm surface, palm up. Palmaris longus tendon can be seen by wrist flexion against resistance.
- Insert the needle at the distal skin crease, at 45° to the horizontal, pointing towards the fingers, just ulnar (little-finger side) to the palmaris tendon. Figure 5.3.
- Use a green (21 gauge) needle and advance it to about ½ its length. If there is sudden pain in the fingers you have hit the median nerve – withdraw the needle and reposition it.
- Inject steroid e.g. 10mg triamcinolone – if there is resistance the needle is not in the right place. Don't use LA as it causes finger numbness.
- Rest the hand for several days afterwards.

🅘 Palmaris longus is absent in 10% – inject between the tendons of flexor digitorum superficialis and flexor carpi radialis.

⚠ Pain may worsen after injection for up to 48h. before it improves – warn the patient.

Elbow: Tennis or golfer's elbow responds well to steroid injection. Steroid is infiltrated into the tender spots at the tendon insertion rather than into a joint space. Thus there is resistance on injection and it can be quite painful – warn the patient.

Technique
- Sit the patient with the elbow flexed to 90o and palpate the most tender spot.
- Insert the needle into that spot and inject 0.1–0.2ml of steroid (e.g. hydrocortisone 25mg/1ml). Then without making a new skin puncture move the needle in a fan shape around the area, injecting small amounts of steroid – try to inject all the tender area – Figure 5.4.
- Pain of injection may last 48h. – advise resting the arm and analgesia.

⚠ The steroid is injected relatively superficially, so warn the patient about the possibility of skin dimpling or pigment loss.

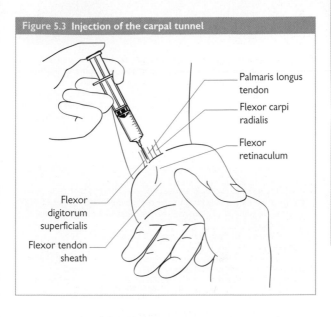

Figure 5.3 Injection of the carpal tunnel

Palmaris longus
tendon

Flexor carpi
radialis

Flexor
retinaculum

Flexor
digitorum
superficialis

Flexor tendon
sheath

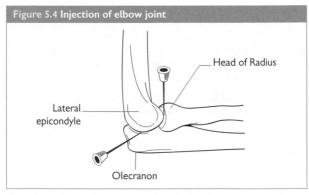

Figure 5.4 Injection of elbow joint

Head of Radius

Lateral
epicondyle

Olecranon

175

Reproduced with permission from the Oxford Handbook of Clinical Specialities (1999),
Oxford University Press, Oxford.

Shoulder: Injection can help rotator cuff problems, frozen shoulder, subacromial bursitis and rheumatoid arthritis. Injection can be located into either the subacromial space or shoulder joint (Figure 5.5). Use an anterior or posterior approach for shoulder joint injection and lateral approach for the subacromial space. The joint space only communicates with the subacromial space if there is a rotator cuff tear – in which case steroid will reach the whole joint whichever approach is used.

Technique: Anterior approach:
- Sit patient with the arm relaxed at the side and slightly externally rotated. Palpate the space between the head of humerus and the coracoid process.
- Insert the needle (green, 21 gauge) horizontally into that gap, ensuring the needle is lateral to the coracoid process – Figure 5.5(a). The needle will need to be inserted for most of its length to reach the joint space.
- Typical dose is 1ml steroid e.g. triamcinolone 20mg + 1ml 1% lidocaine.
- There should be no/little resistance to injecting the fluid – if there is, the needle is wrongly positioned.

Technique: *Lateral approach to subacromial space*
- Sit patient with arm hanging down to the side
- Palpate the postero-lateral corner of the acromion
- Insert the needle horizontally into the space beneath the acromion – Figure 5.5(b)
- Use 5ml 0.5% marcaine + triamcinolone 20μg

AC joint injection: Can help the pain of OA.

Technique
- Palpate the joint space – the needle can be inserted anteriorly or superiorly. If you push the needle too far you may enter the shoulder joint (Figure 5.5(c)).
- Small joint space means only 0.2–0.5ml can be injected.
- Use a blue (23 gauge) needle and don't add LA.

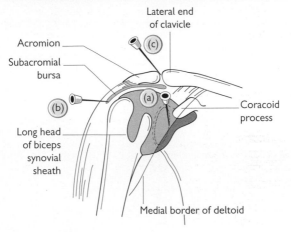

Figure 5.5 Injection of shoulder joint

Lateral end of clavicle

Acromion

Subacromial bursa

(b)

Long head of biceps synovial sheath

(a)

(c)

Coracoid process

Medial border of deltoid

(a) Anterior approach joint injection
(b) Subacromial space injection
(c) Acromioclavicular joint injection

Reproduced with modifications from the Oxford Handbook of Clinical Specialties (1999). Oxford University Press, Oxford.

Chapter 6

Benefits and support available for people with musculoskeletal problems and their carers

Benefits

⚠️ Information in this section is up to date at the time of going to press but benefits issues change rapidly.

Millions of pounds of benefits go unclaimed every year. This chapter is a rough guide to the benefits available to enable GPs to point their patients in the right direction. It is not intended as a comprehensive reference.

Agency	Function	Website: www. + suffix	Telephone
Table 6.1 Guide to agencies involved in delivering benefits to patients			
Department of Work and Pensions (DWP)	Administers all benefits *except:* Tax credits (Inland Revenue) Statutory sick pay (employer) Housing benefit (local authority) Council tax benefit (local authority)	dwp.gov.uk	*Benefits Enquiry Line –* 0800 882200 *Help with form completion –* 0800 441144 *Information for employers and the self-employed –* 0845 7143143
Jobcentre Plus	Helps people of working age to find work and get any benefits they are entitled to	jobcentreplus.gov.uk	Contact local office (list available on website)
Pension Service	Provides services and support for pensioners and people looking into pensions and retirement	thepension service.gov.uk	Contact area office (list available on website)
Inland Revenue	Administers tax credits	hmrc.gov.uk	Tax credit enquiry line – 0845 300 3900
Disability and Carers Service	Delivers a range of benefits to disabled people and their carers	disability.gov.uk	Contact local disability benefits office (list available on DWP website)
Appeals Service	Provides an independent tribunal body for hearing appeals	appeals-service.gov.uk	N/A

ℹ️ 0800 numbers are free; 0845 numbers are charged at local rate

> ⚠ **Benefit fraud:** The DWP provides a freefone number which members of the public can telephone in confidence to give information about benefit fraud. ☎ 0800 85 44 40

Further information for health professionals
Department of Work and Pensions (DWP): 🖥 www.dwp.gov.uk

Further information for patients and carers
Government information and services: 🖥 www.direct.gov.uk
Citizens' Advice Bureau: 🖥 www.adviceguide.org.uk
Age Concern: ☎ 0800 00 99 66 🖥 www.ageconcern.org.uk
Help the Aged: ☎ 0800 800 65 65 🖥 www.helptheaged.org.uk
Counsel and Care: ☎ 0845 300 7585 🖥 www.counselandcare.org.uk

Pensions

War pensions: For people injured whilst serving in the armed forces and their dependants (if injury caused or hastened death). Administered by the Veterans Agency, MoD. No time limit for claims. *Benefits:*

War disablement pension
- *Basic benefits:* Based on percentage disablement:
  - If <20% disabled – lump sum
  - If >20% disabled – weekly sum (pension)
- *Other benefits:* Allowances if severely disabled e.g.:
  - War pensioners mobility supplement – for walking difficulty. Holders can apply for the motability scheme and road tax exemption.
  - Constant attendance allowance – for high levels of care.

Medical treatment: Some services and appliances may be paid for by the Veterans Agency (includes prescription charges, nursing home fees).

War widows' and widowers' pensions: Payable if spouse's death was as a result of service or, in certain circumstances, if spouse received a war pension prior to death.

Veterans Agency: ☎ 0800 169 22 77
🖥 www.veteransagency.mod.uk

Retirement pension: A state retirement pension is payable to women aged ≥60y. and men aged ≥65y., even if still working. Claim forms should be received automatically – if not request one through the local Jobcentre Plus office. Pensions are taxable.

Basic pension: Flat rate amount – different for single people and married couples. If not enough national insurance (NI) contributions have been paid amounts may ↓. >80y. higher rate payable which is not dependent on NI contributions.

Increase for dependants: Paid if:
- The claimant's spouse is <60y. and earns under a set amount/does not receive certain other benefits.
- The claimant has children (if claim made before April 2003).

Additional pension: State second pension (replaced SERPS). Based on NI contributions and earnings. Workers can opt out of the additional pension scheme, pay into a private or company scheme instead and pay lower NI.

Graduated pension: Some people may be entitled to a graduated pension. This is based on earnings between 1961 and 1975.

Extra pension: For a person who defers claiming retirement pension for up to 5y. Extra pension is payable when retirement pension is claimed.

❶ If hospitalized, retirement pension is payable for 1y. at full rate. After 12mo., basic pension is ↓ but additional pension stays the same.

Other benefits for pensioners
- *Pension credit:* 📖 p.184
- *Free colour television licence:* All pensioners >75y.
- *Winter fuel payment:* Annual payment to all pensioners >60y.
  Freephone advice service: ☎ 0800 22 44 88
- *Cold weather payment:* 📖 p.186

Home Responsibilities Protection (HRP): Scheme which protects basic state pension for people who don't work or have low income and are caring for someone. 🖥 www.thepensionservice.gov.uk

Christmas bonus: One-off payment made to people receiving a retirement pension or income support a few weeks before Christmas.

Table 6.2 Benefits for people with low income

	Eligibility	How to apply	Benefits gained
Income Support (IS)	• ≥18y. (16y. in some circumstances) and <60y. • Low income, <£8000 in savings (£16,000 if in residential care) and not in receipt of JSA • <16h. paid work/wk. (and partner <24h./wk.)	Form A1 from local Jobcentre Plus office	*Money* – depends on circumstances *Other benefits* – housing benefit, community tax benefit, health benefits and Social Fund payments. Children <5y. and pregnant women – free milk and vitamins. Children >5y. – free school meals and, in some areas, uniform grants *Christmas bonus* – 📖 p.183
Job Seeker's Allowance (JSA)	• ≥19y. and <60y. (women) or <65y. (men) • Unemployed or working <16h./wk. • Capable of and available for work • Have a Job Seeker's agreement that contracts the recipient to actively seek work	Apply by visiting local job centre	*Contributions-based JSA* – can claim for up to 26wk. Age-dependent fixed weekly payment *Income-based JSA* – allowance dependent on circumstances. Entitles claimants to same benefits as Income Support (see above) *Hardship payment* – available to people disallowed JSA
Pension credit	*Guarantee credit:* ≥60y. and income below the 'appropriate amount'. Appropriate amount varies according to circumstances. Capital (excluding value of own home) >£6000 is deemed to count as income at the rate of £1/wk. /£500 capital *Savings credit:* ≥65y. and income > savings credit starting point – currently >£114.05/wk. for a single person or >£174.05 if one of a couple. Depends on level of income and circumstances	Apply on form PC1 ☎ 0800 991234	*Money* – depends on circumstances *Other benefits* – if receiving guarantee credit automatically eligible for housing benefit, community tax benefit and Social Fund payments

Working Tax Credit (WTC)	• Age ≥16y., working ≥16h./wk. and responsible for a child (<16y. or 16–19y. in full-time education) • Age ≥16y., working ≥16h./wk. and has a disability • Age ≥50y., working ≥16h./wk. and has started work after ≥6mo. of receiving 1 of certain benefits • Age ≥25y. and working ≥30h./wk.	Apply to Inland Revenue ☎ 0845 300 3900 🖳 www.hmrc.gov.uk	*Tax credits* – depends on adding together elements: • Basic element – paid to everyone entitled to WTC • Second adult element • Lone parent element • Working >30h./wk. (can combine both parents if have children) • Disability (if working >16h./wk.) • Severe disability (if working >16h./wk.) • Aged ≥50y. and in receipt of certain benefits before resuming work • Childcare – up to 70% childcare costs
Children's Tax Credit (CTC)	• Age ≥16y. and • Responsible for ≥1 child (<16y. or 16–19y. and in full-time education) • Family income <£50,000 pa	Apply to Inland Revenue ☎ 0845 300 3900 🖳 www.hmrc.gov.uk	*Tax credits:* • Family element – credit for any family, eligible – if there is a child <1y. old in the family • Child element – credit for each individual child in the family – if the child is disabled/severely disabled
Health benefits	Automatic entitlement: • Age >60y. or <16y. (19y. if in full-time education) • Claiming IS or income-based JSA • Pregnant or within 1y. of childbirth By application: • Low income and • Savings <£8000	If automatic exemption, no need to claim. If not, claim using form HC1, available from pharmacies, GP surgeries and local Jobcentre Plus offices	*Free:* • Prescriptions • NHS dentistry • NHS eye tests and glasses • NHS wigs and fabric supports • Travel to hospital • Milk and vitamins for pregnant and breast-feeding women, and children <5y.

Table 6.2 Benefits for people with low income (Contd.)

	Eligibility	How to apply	Benefits gained
Housing benefit	Low income, living in rented housing *Exclusions:* Full-time students without dependants, people in residential care or with savings >£16,000	Via local authority	Pays rent for up to 60wk, then need to reapply
Council tax benefit and Second adult rebate	• Council tax benefit – low income. Exclusions as for housing benefit • Second adult rebate: payable if someone who lives with you is aged >18y, does not pay rent or council tax and has low income • Council tax reduction – if single occupier or disabled • Disregarded occupants – certain people, including students, carers and children, are not counted in calculating the number of people living at a property	Via local authority	Council tax benefit – pays council tax Council tax reductions: • single occupier – 25% discount • all disregarded occupants – 50% • disabled – reduction to next lowest council tax band
The 6 social Fund payments	• Crisis loan – anyone except students and people in residential care can apply • Budgeting loan – for large purchases. Must receive IS, pension credit or income-based JSA • Funeral payments – must receive low income benefit and be responsible for the funeral • Cold weather payments – average temperature <0°C for ≥7d. Must receive IS, pension credit or income-based JSA and live with a pensioner, child <5y, or disabled person • Maternity grant • Community care grant – 🕮 p.187	Cold weather payments – should be automatic All others claim via local Jobcentre Plus offices or 🖳 www.dwp.gov.uk	• Crisis loan – up to £1000 – interest-free loan, repayable when crisis finished over 78wk. • Budgeting loan – as crisis loan • Funeral expenses – sum towards cost of funeral – usually does not cover full expenses • Cold weather payments – £8.50/wk.

Table 6.3 Benefits for disability and illness

	Eligibility	How to apply	Amount
Statutory Sick Pay	• Employee age ≥16y. and <65y. • Incapable of work due to sickness or disability • Earning ≥ NI lower earnings limit • Unable to work ≥4d. and <28wk. (inc. days when would not normally work) • Those ineligible may be eligible for Incapacity Benefit or Maternity Allowance	Notify employer of illness – self-certification first 7d. (SC2); Med 3 after that time	£68.20/wk. Some employers have more generous arrangements. Paid through normal pay mechanisms
Incapacity Benefit	• Not entitled to Statutory Sick Pay (includes self-employed) • Unable to work (Med 3 certification until Personal Capability Assessment is applied when GP may be asked for short factual report or Med 4.) • < pensionable age • Sufficient NI contributions (unless aged <20y.)	Form SC1 available from GP surgeries, hospitals and local social security offices. If employed and unable to claim SSP apply on form SSP1 supplied by employer	1–28 weeks – £59.20/wk. 29–52 weeks – £70.05/wk. >52 weeks – £78.50/wk. Plus additions for dependants. A higher rate is payable if <45y. when became unable to work or if over state retirement age
Community Care Grant	Receiving Income Support or income-based Jobseeker's Allowance and: • to re-establish or help the applicant or a family member stay in the community • to ease exceptional pressure on the applicant or a family member • to help with certain travel costs	Form SF300 from local social security offices or ⏵ www.dwp.gov.uk	Minimum payment £30. No maximum amount
Disabled Facilities Grant	For work essential to help a disabled person live an independent life. Means tested	Apply via local housing department	Any reasonable application for funds is considered

187

Table 6.3 Benefits for disability and illness (Contd.)

	Eligibility	How to apply	Amount
Disability Living Allowance (DLA)▽	• Disability >3mo. and expected to last >6 mo. more* • <65y. at time of application Mobility component: Help needed to get about outdoors • Higher rate – unable/virtually unable to walk (age >3y.) • Lower rate – help to find way in unfamiliar places (age >5y.) Care component: Help needed with personal care • Lower rate – attention/supervision needed for a significant proportion of the day or unable to prepare a cooked meal • Middle rate – attention/supervision throughout the day or repeated prolonged attention or watching over at night • Higher rate – 24-hour attention/supervision or terminal illness*	☎ 0800 882200 (0800 220674 in Northern Ireland) or Leaflet DS704 available from post offices or Using claim packs available at CAB and social security offices or 🖥 www.dwp.gov.uk	Mobility component: Higher rate – £43.45/wk. Lower rate – £16.50/wk. Care component: Higher rate – £62.25/wk. Middle rate – £41.65/wk. Lower rate – £16.50/wk.
Attendance Allowance (AA)▽	• Disability >3mo. and expected to last >6 mo. more* • Aged ≥65y. • Not permanently in hospital or accommodation funded by the local authority • Needs attention/supervision – higher rate if 24-hour care required/terminal illness*	☎ 0800 882200 (0800 220674 in Northern Ireland) or Leaflet DS704 available from Post Offices or 🖥 www.dwp.gov.uk	Lower rate – £41.65/wk. Higher rate – £62.25/wk. (for people who need day and night care or are terminally ill)

▽ No need to receive help to apply. Not means tested.

* Terminal illness (not expected to live >6mo.) – claim under Special Rules. Claims are processed much faster and the highest care rate is automatically awarded. GP or hospital specialist fills in form DS1500 to provide clinical information to support application (fee can be claimed).

| Carer's Allowance | • Aged ≥16y.; and
• Spends ≥35h./wk. caring for a person with a disability who is getting AA or Constant Attendance Allowance or middle or higher rate care component of DLA; and
• Earning ≤£84.00/wk., after allowable expenses
• Not in full-time education | Complete form in leaflet DS700, available from local social security offices or 🖥 www.dwp.gov.uk | £46.95/wk.
Plus additions for dependants.
(ℹ No new claims for dependent children have accepted since April 2003) |

ℹ
• People who need someone's help to get out of the house are entitled to free prescriptions.
• *Severe Disablement Allowance* is still paid to those who applied prior to April 2001.

Table 6.4 Mobility for disabled and elderly people ● Local public transport schemes also exist

	Eligibility	How to apply	Benefits gained
Blue Badge Scheme	Age >2y, and ≥1 of the following: ● War pension mobility supplement ● Higher rate of the mobility component of DLA ● Motor vehicle supplied by a government health department ● Registered blind ● Severe disability in both upper limbs preventing turning of a steering wheel ● Permanent and substantial difficulty walking	Apply through local social services department ● In most circumstances the disabled person does not have to be the driver. The badge should not be used if the disabled person is not in the car 🖳 www.dft.gov.uk	Entitles holder to park: ● in specified disabled spaces ● free of charge or time limit at parking meters or other places where waiting is limited ● on single yellow lines for up to 3h. (no time limit in Scotland)
Motability Scheme	● Higher rate mobility component of DLA or ● War pension mobility supplement ● Driver may be someone else	Contact Motability. Application guide available at 🖳 www.motability.co.uk	Registered charity. Mobility payments can be used to lease or hire-purchase a car, powered scooter or wheelchair. Grants may also be available for advance payments, adaptations or driving lessons
Road tax exemption	● Higher rate mobility component of DLA or ● War pension mobility supplement or ● Person nominated as someone who regularly drives for a disabled person or ● Certain types of powered invalid carriages	Usually received automatically. If not and claiming DLA, ☎ 0845 712 3456. If claiming war pension, ☎ 0800 169 2277	Exemption from road tax
Seatbelt exemption	Certain medical conditions e.g. colostomy	Medical practitioner must complete exemption certificate	Exemption from wearing seatbelt

Table 6.5 Adaptations and equipment for disabled and elderly people ● All purchases related to disability are VAT exempt

	Eligibility	Applying	Benefits received
Wheelchairs	Anyone requiring a wheelchair(s) for >3mo. Short-term loan of equipment is often available via the Red Cross	Referral by GP or specialist to wheelchair service centre. Directory service centres available at: ⌨ www.wheelchairmanagers.nhs.uk	Provision of suitable wheelchair. Vouchers enable disabled patients to purchase their chairs privately
Occupational therapy (OT) assessment	All elderly or disabled people	Request needs assessment by occupational therapist via local social services department	Enables provision of equipment and adaptations necessary to maintain an independent lifestyle
Disabled Living Centres/Disability Living Foundation	All elderly or disabled people	49 Disabled Living Centres in the UK – list available at ⌨ www.dlcc.co.uk Disabled Living Foundation: ⌨ www.dlf.org.uk. ☎ 0845 130 9177	Disabled Living Centres – look at and try out equipment, with OTs on hand to advise Disabled Living Foundation – information on aids and adaptations
Telephone	People who have physical difficulty using the telephone or communication problems	British Telecom produce a booklet 'Communication Solutions', obtainable from ☎ 0800 800150 or ⌨ www.bt.com If difficulty using a telephone directory, register to use directory enquiries free ☎ 0800 5870195	Gadgets and services that make it easier for disabled or elderly people to use the telephone.
Alarm systems	Any disabled or elderly person who is alone at times, at risk, and mentally capable of using an alarm system	Arrange via local social services or housing department. Alternatively charities for the elderly have schemes (Help the Aged – seniorlink ☎ 01255 473 999; Age Concern – Aid-Call ☎ 0800 772266)	Enables a call for help when the phone cannot be reached

Criminal injury and occupational illness

Criminal injuries: Compensation may be available for victims of violent crimes, even if the attacker is not identified. Compensation is paid for the injury, loss of earnings and expenses. Contact Criminal Injuries Compensation Authority 🖥 www.cica.gov.uk

Occupational illness: If a patient develops an occupational disease, a doctor is obliged to notify their employer in writing with the patient's consent. The doctor does not need to make a judgment about whether the disease is, in that particular case, caused by the occupation.

Employers must then inform the Reporting of Injuries, Diseases and Dangerous Occurrences Regulations (RIDDOR) incident contact centre (☎ 0845 300 99 23 🖥 www.riddor.gov.uk). Self-employed patients must contact RIDDOR themselves.

Patients who do not give consent for the doctor to notify their employer may allow the doctor to inform the employer's occupational health department or RIDDOR directly instead.

Notifiable industrial diseases:	🛈 This is not a complete list
• Poisoning by industrial agents e.g. lead, arsenic, mercury	• Chrome ulceration
• Repetitive strain injury	• Tenosynovitis e.g. as a result of repeated movements of the hand/wrist
• Vibration white finger	• Pneumoconiosis
• Bursitis e.g. housemaid's knee	• Extrinsic allergic alveolitis
• Occupational asthma	• Occupational deafness
• Folliculitis and acne (associated with work with tar, pitch or oils)	• Occupational cancers e.g. nasopharyngeal cancer in woodworkers; bladder cancer in plastic workers; cancers as a result of ionizing radiation; mesothelioma due to asbestos
• Occupational infection e.g. hepatitis B in health care workers, anthrax in farmers	
• Irritant dermatitis e.g. hairdressers' dermatitis	

192

Industrial injury: Injured employees should always report details of the accident – however trivial the injury – to their employer and record them in the accident book as soon as possible. Employers must inform RIDDOR of:
• dangerous incidents – even if no one was hurt
• incidents where death or serious injury occurs
• incidents resulting in injury requiring >3d. absence from work
• incidents involving gas.

Prescribed industrial disease: Disease for which benefit is paid if the applicant worked in a job for which that disease is 'prescribed' and it is likely the employment caused the disease. Claims may be made at any time with the exceptions of occupational deafness (claim <5y. after leaving employment) and occupational asthma (claim <10y. after leaving employment). The list of prescribed diseases is similar to but *not* the same as the list of notifiable diseases.

Benefits payable

Industrial Injuries Disablement Benefit: Available to:
- A person in paid employment at the time of the accident or when s/he contracted the disease;
- If the injury is as a result of an accident or certain (prescribed) illness arising as a result of employment, even if the employee was either part or wholly to blame; *and*

If disability is assessed at ≥14% (exceptions: occupational deafness >20%; dust-related lung disease – no level).Industrial covers virtually all forms of work. If a patient claims benefit for >1 industrial accident or disease, assessments may be added together and benefit awarded on the total.

For accidents, claims can be made at any time after the event but benefit is paid only if there are still effects of the injury after the 91st day.

Reduced Earnings Allowance: Accident occurred/disease contracted prior to 1st October 1990, disablement assessment of ≥1%; *and*
- unable to work; *or*
- unable to work at normal job; *or*
- working less hours at normal job.

Retirement Allowance: Reduced Earnings Allowance becomes Retirement Allowance at age 60y. (♀) or 65y. (♂). It is paid at 25% the rate of Reduced Earnings Allowance when a claimant stopped work.

Constant Attendance Allowance: For people so disabled they need constant care and attention and who are getting disablement benefit for disability assessed at 100%. 4 rates of benefit.

Exceptionally Severe Disablement Allowance: For people who get constant attendance allowance at high rate and where need for attendance is likely to be permanent.

🛈 People who suffer from industrial diseases or have suffered disability as a result of an industrial accident are also eligible to apply for benefits available for any disabled individuals – 📖 pp.187–9.

Making claims: Through local Jobcentre Plus or social security office. A full list of prescribed industrial diseases is also available from these places. Some claims can be made online 🖥 www.jobcentreplus. gov.uk

Useful contacts
RIDDOR – incident contact centre: ☎ 0845 300 99 23
🖥 www.riddor.gov.uk
Health and Safety Executive: ☎ 0870 1545500
🖥 www.hse.gov.uk
Jobcentre Plus: 🖥 www.jobcentreplus.gov.uk
Trade Unions

Chapter 7

The General Medical Services contract and musculoskeletal problems

The General Medical Services (GMS) contract

Although there may be some differences in process in each of the four countries of the UK, the principles of the GMS contract apply to all. A total sum for GMS services is given to each primary care organization (PCO) as part of a bigger unified budget allocation. PCOs are responsible for managing the GMS budget locally.

The contract: Made between an individual practice and a PCO. All the partners of the practice, at least one of whom must be a GP, have to sign the contract. It includes:
- National terms applicable to all practices (the 'practice contract')
- Which services will be provided by that practice i.e.
  - essential
  - additional – if not opted out
  - out-of-hours – if not opted out
  - enhanced – if opted in
- Level of quality of essential and additional services that the practice 'aspires' to
- Support arrangements e.g. IT, premises
- Total financial resources i.e. global sum + quality achievement payments + enhanced services payments + premises + IT + dispensing.

Essential services: All practices must undertake these services. *Include:*
- *Day-to-day medical care of the practice population:* health promotion, management of minor and self-limiting illness and referral to secondary care services and other agencies as appropriate
- *General management of patients who are terminally ill*
- *Chronic disease management*

Additional services: Services the practice will usually undertake but may 'opt out' of. If the practice opts out, the PCO takes responsibility for providing the service instead. The practice then receives a ↓ global sum payment.

Enhanced services: Commissioned by the PCO and paid for *in addition* to the global sum payment. 3 types:
- *Directed enhanced services:* services under national direction with national specifications and benchmark pricing which all PCOs must commission to cover their relevant population.
- *National enhanced services:* services with national minimum standards and benchmark pricing but not directed (i.e. PCOs do not have to provide these services).
- *Services developed locally* to meet local needs (local enhanced services) e.g. enhanced care of the homeless.

Table 7.1 Payment under the GMS contract

Payment	Explanation
The global sum	Major part of the money paid to practices. Paid monthly and intended to cover practice running costs. *Includes provision for:* • Delivery of essential services and additional/out-of-hours services if not opted out • Staff costs • Career development • Locum reimbursement (e.g. for appraisal, career development, and protected time).
Aspiration payments	Advance payments to allow practices to develop services to achieve higher quality standards. Aspiration payments are made monthly alongside global sum payments and amount to roughly 60% of the points achieved in the previous year (for 2005/6 this was ≈ 2004/5 points achieved × £ 124.60/ points ×60% × last size and composition adjustment).
Achievement payments	Payments made for the practice's achieved number of points in the quality and outcomes framework (📖 p.198), as measured at the start of the following year. Aspiration payments already received are deducted from the total i.e. payment for actual points less aspiration pay.
Payment for 'extra' services	Paid to practices that provide directed enhanced services, national enhanced services and/or local enhanced services to meet local needs.
Minimum practice income guarantee (MPIG)	Protects those practices that lost out under the redistribution effect of the new resource allocation formula. Calculated from the difference between the global sum allocation (GSA) under the new GMS contract and the global sum equivalent (GSE) – the amount the practice would have earned for providing the same service under the old GMS contract ('The Red Book'). If GSA < GSE, a correction factor (CF) will be applied as long as necessary so that GSA+CF=GSE.
Other payments	Payments for premises, IT and dispensing (dispensing practices only).

❶ The Carr-Hill allocation formula is a GMS resource allocation formula for allocating funds for the global sum and quality payments. The formula takes the practice population and then makes a series of adjustments based on the profile of the local community, taking account of determinants of relative practice workload and costs.

The quality and outcomes framework

The quality and outcomes framework (QOF) was developed specifically for the new GMS contract. Financial incentives are used to encourage high-quality care.

The domains: The GMS quality framework is divided into 4 domains:
- Clinical
- Organizational
- Additional services
- Patient experience

See Table 7.2

Indicators: Every domain has a set of 'indicators' which relate to quality standards or guidelines that can be achieved within that domain. The indicators were developed by an expert group based on the best available evidence at the time and will be updated regularly. All data should be obtainable from practice clinical systems and Read codes have been developed to make this easier. Indicators are split into 3 types:
- *Structure* e.g. is a disease register in place?
- *Process:* e.g. is a particular measure being recorded? Is action being taken where appropriate?
- *Outcome:* e.g. how well is the condition being controlled?

Quality points: All achievement against quality indicators converts to points. Each point has a monetary value.
- *Yes/no indicators:* All points are allocated if the result is +ve and none if -ve.
- *Range of attainment:* For most of clinical indicators it is not possible to attain 100% results (even if allowed exceptions are applied) so a range of satisfactory attainment is specified. Minimum standard is 40%. Points are allocated in a linear fashion based on comparison with attainment against a maximum standard e.g. if the maximum % for an indicator is 90%, the minimum 40% and the practice achieves 70%, the practice will receive 30/50 (i.e. 3/5) of the available points.

Reporting on quality: Every year each practice must complete a standard return form recording level of achievement and the evidence for that. In addition there is an annual quality review visit by the PCO. Based on these, the PCO confirms level of achievement funding attained and discusses points the practice will 'aspire' to the following year (🕮 p.197). The process is confirmed in writing by the PCO and signed off by the practice. The Commission for Healthcare Audit and Inspection (or equivalents in Scotland/NI) checks quality countrywide.

The quality framework and the Personal Medical Services (PMS) contract: Mechanisms for quality delivery and the quality framework are broadly comparable for GMS and PMS practices. PMS practices can apply for aspiration payments and achievement payments in the same way as GMS practices. However, in order to reflect the local nature of the contracts, standards PMS practices are working to do not have to be the same as those contained in the National Quality Framework. Nevertheless, all standards must be: rigorous; evidence based; monitored fairly; assessed against criteria agreed between PCOs and providers; and paid at appropriate and equitable rates.

Table 7.2 Calculation of points for quality framework payments

Components of total points score	Points	Way in which points are calculated
Clinical indicators	655	Achieving pre-set standards in management of: • Smoking • Dementia • Palliative care • Learning difficulty • CHD • Depression • Left ventricular dysfunction • Mental health • Atrial fibrillation • COPD • Stroke and TIA • Asthma • Hypertension • Epilepsy • Hypothyroidism • Cancer • DM • Obesity • Chronic kidney disease
Organizational	181	Achieving pre-set standards in: • Records and information about patients • Information for patients • Education and training • Medicines management • Practice management
Additional services	36	Achieving pre-set standards in: • Cervical screening • Child health surveillance • Maternity services • Contraceptive services
Patient experience	108	Achieving pre-set standards in: • Patient survey* • Consultation length
Holistic care	200	Reflects range of achievement across clinical indicators – calculated by ranking clinical indicators in terms of proportion of points gained (1–10). Proportion of the points gained by the 3rd lowest indicator (i.e. indicator ranked 7) is the proportion of the holistic care points obtained.
Total possible	1000	

In 2005/6 and 2006/7 the average value of 1 point = £124.60

*Improving Patient Questionnaire (IPQ – charge payable) –
🖳 www.cfep.co.uk or General Practice Assessment Questionnaire (GPAQ) –
🖳 www.gpaq.info

Further information

DoH: *The GMS Contract.* 🖳 www.dh.gov.uk
BMA: *The blue book and supporting documents.* 🖳 www.bma.org.uk

Relevant quality indicators

Medication: Many patients with chronic musculoskeletal problems take medication over long periods of time. They are often cared for by a multidisciplinary team with more than one agency initiating and pre-scribing medication. *It is important that:*

- The medicines the patient is receiving are clearly listed on their record (Records 7)
- The record of medication is kept up to date – whichever team member is involved (Records 12) and that the notes have a clear indication of when the drug was started and what it was prescribed for (Records 9)
- Any drug allergies or adverse reactions are clearly recorded (Records 8)
- Regular review of repeat medication is carried out (Medicines 11 and 12).

Carers: Many patients with chronic musculoskeletal problems are looked after by informal carers (📖 p.166). As a result of their caring role, many carers develop physical and mental health problems. Indenti-fying and supporting them (Management 9) can help maintain carer health and keep patients in the community longer.

Table 7.3 Summary of relevant indicators

Indicator	Description	Points	Payment stages
Records 8	There is a designated place for the recording of drug allergies and adverse reactions in the notes and these are clearly recorded	1 point	
Records 9	For repeat medicines, an indication for the drug can be identified in the records (for drugs added to the repeat prescription with effect from 1 April 2004)	4 points	Minimum standard 80%
Management 9	The practice has a protocol for the identification of carers and a mechanism for the referral of carers for social services assessment	3 points	
Medicines 11	A medication review is recorded in the notes in the preceding 15 months for all patients being prescribed 4 or more repeat medicines	7 points	Minimum standard 80%
Medicines 12	A medication review is recorded in the notes in the preceding 15 months for all patients being prescribed repeat medicines	8 points	Minimum standard 80%

Relevant additional and directed enhanced services

Minor surgery as an additional service: Includes curettage and cautery and, in relation to warts, verrucae and other skin lesions, cryo-cautery. In all cases a record of consent of the patient to treatment and a record of the procedure itself should be kept. Payment is included within the global sum payment. If a practice does not want to provide this service it must 'opt out' and global sum payment is ↓ by 0.6%.

Minor surgery as a directed enhanced service: Extends the range of procedures beyond those practices are expected to do as an additional service. For the purpose of payment, procedures have been divided into 3 groups:
- Injections – muscles, tendons and joints
- Invasive procedures – including incisions and excisions
- Injections of varicose veins and piles.

Payment: Treatments are priced according to the complexity of the procedure, involvement of other staff and use of specialized equipment. Terms for this must be negotiated locally. Typical figures in 2004/5 are £40 for a joint injection or £80 for a simple excision.

Qualification to provide the service: Practices can provide this service if they can demonstrate they have the necessary facilities and personnel (partner, employee or sub-contractor) with the necessary skills. *This includes:*
- Adequate equipment
- Premises compliant with national guidelines as contained in Health Building note 46: General medical practice premises (DoH)
- Nursing support
- Compliance with national infection control policies – sterile packs from the local CSSD, disposable sterile instruments, using approved sterilization procedures etc.
- Ongoing training in minor surgery, related skills and resuscitation techniques
- Regular audit and peer review to monitor clinical outcomes, rates of infection and procedure.

Minor surgery in PMS practices: PMS contracts are negotiated on an individual basis with the local PCO. In most cases, however, the contract provides for similar arrangements and payments to those in place for GMS practices.

GMS contract		
Management Indicator 4	The arrangements for instrument sterilization comply with national guidelines as applicable to primary care	1 point

Influenza and pneumococcal immunizations for at-risk groups as a directed enhanced service: This directed enhanced service aims to provide influenza and pneumococcal vaccination for the elderly and other 'at-risk' groups, including those taking immuno-suppressant drugs for arthritis. Practices DO NOT have preferred provider status for this service.

Target group for influenza vaccination
- Patients aged ≥65y. at the end of the financial year
- Patients suffering from chronic respiratory disease (including asthma), chronic heart disease, chronic liver disease, chronic renal disease, immunosuppression due to disease or treatment, or diabetes mellitus
- Patients living in long-stay residential or nursing homes or other long-stay health or social care facilities
- Carers of people with chronic disabilities

Target group for pneumococcal vaccination
- Patients ≥65y. at the end of the financial year
- Patients suffering from chronic respiratory disease (including asthma), chronic heart disease, chronic renal disease or nephrotic syndrome, chronic liver disease including cirrhosis, immunosuppression due to disease or treatment (including HIV infection at all stages), asplenia or severe dysfunction of the spleen (including homozygous sickle cell disease and coeliac disease), diabetes mellitus, or individuals with CSF shunts
- Children <5y. who have previously had invasive pneumococcal disease
- Patients living in long-stay residential or nursing homes or other long-stay health or social care facilities

Qualifications to provide the service
- Practices are expected to use a call – recall system identifying those 'at risk' through existing registers compiled for use within the quality and outcomes framework.
- Practices not participating in the quality and outcomes framework must compile a register to qualify to provide this enhanced service.

Targets
- No target has been set for the proportion of 'at-risk' patients given pneumococcal vaccination.
- A target of 70% has been set for influenza vaccination of patients ≥65y. However, a fee per vaccination is payable whether or not this target is reached.
- Additional payments are available through the quality and outcomes framework for vaccinating high proportions of 'at-risk' patients against influenza.

National enhanced services

These are services with national minimum standards and benchmark pricing but are not 'directed' (i.e. PCOs do not have to provide these services).

Provision of near-patient testing

This national enhanced service will fund a shared-care-drug monitoring service in respect of the following drugs:

- Penicillamine
- Auranofin
- Sulphasalazine
- Methotrexate
- Sodium aurothiomalate.

And all other 'amber' list drugs where shared care is appropriate.

Practices providing this service must

- Maintain a register of patients being monitored including name, date of birth, indication and duration of treatment and last hospital appointment
- Provide a call – recall system
- Educate newly diagnosed patients and provide ongoing information for established patients
- Create an individual management plan for each patient on the register
- Work together with other professionals and refer on where necessary
- Keep records of the service provided including all information relating to significant events e.g. hospital admission, death
- Provide ongoing training to staff involved
- Review the scheme annually including internal and external quality assurance for any computer-aided decision-making equipment or near-patient testing equipment used.

🔔 Practitioners must notify the PCO clinical governance lead:
- *of any emergency admission* due to usage of the drug(s) in question or attributable to the relevant underlying medical condition of a patient covered by this service
- *of any death* due to usage of the drug(s) in question or attributable to the relevant underlying medical condition of a patient covered by this service
- *<72h. after learning of the event.*

Fees vary according to whether:
- *the blood is taken in the practice or not*
- *the sample is tested in the practice or not, and*
- *the dose is monitored by the practice or not.*

4 levels of payment. Scale of fees is £6–120/patient/y. In addition a fee of £3–5 per home visit for testing is payable.

Minor injury services

This service will fund:

- Premises and equipment necessary to enable proper provision of a minor injuries service
- Nurses to staff the minor injury service
- Maintenance of infection control standards
- Initial triage of minor injury patients
- History taking, relevant examination and documentation (including record of all procedures)
- Information provision to patients on treatment options and treatment proposed
- Wound assessment
- Histological assessment of all tissue removed by minor surgery in these clinics
- Referral and/or follow-up arrangements
- Regular review of the service including audit and patient feedback.

🚫 Doctors providing this service must be suitably qualified.

Funding available: £1000/year + £50/patient episode. All drugs, dressings and appliances are funded separately by the PCO.

Chapter 8

Useful information and contacts for GPs and patients

Useful information and contacts for GPs

General information

Arthritis Research Campaign (ARC) ☎ 0870 850 5000
🖳 www.arc.org.uk

British Society for Rheumatology 🖳 www.rheumatology.org.uk

Primary Care Rheumatology Society ☎ 01609 774794
🖳 www.pcrsociety.org.uk

Achilles tendon rupture

Bandolier: *Ruptured Achilles tendons – systematic review* (2002)
🖳 www.jr2.ox.ac.uk/bandolier/band103/b103-5.html

Back pain

PRODIGY: *Guidance on lower back pain* 🖳 www.prodigy.nhs.uk

New Zealand Screening Questionnaire for psychosocial barriers to recovery available at 🖳 www.nzgg.org.nz

Child protection

DoH 🖳 www.dh.gov.uk
- *Working together to safeguard children* (1998)
- *What to do if you're worried a child is being abused* (2003)

RCGP: Carter & Bannon. *The role of primary care in the protection of children from abuse and neglect* (2003) 🖳 www.rcgp.org.uk

Department for Education and Skills: *Every child matters* (2004)
🖳 www.everychildmatters.gov.uk

Chronic fatigue syndrome

King's College 🖳 www.kcl.ac.uk/cfs

Royal Australian College of Physicians: *Chronic fatigue syndrome*
🖳 www.mja.com.au/public/guides/cfs/cfs1.html

Fukuda K. *et al.* (1994) The chronic fatigue syndrome: a comprehensive approach to its definition and study. *Annals of Internal Medicine.* 121: 953–9.

Chronic illness

Von Korff *et al.* (2002) Organising care for chronic illness. *BMJ.* 325: 92–4.
🖳 www.bmj.com

Expert Patient Scheme 🖳 www.expertpatients.nhs.uk

Disability and benefits

Department of Work and Pensions (DWP)
🖳 www.dwp.gov.uk

Medical evidence for Statutory Sick Pay, Statutory Maternity Pay and Social Security Incapacity Benefit purposes: a guide for registered medical practitioners. IB204. April 2000.
🖳 www.dwp.gov.uk/medical/medicalib204/index.asp

Disability Discrimination Act 🖳 www.disability.gov.uk

Jobcentre Plus 🖳 www.jobcentreplus.gov.uk

Driving

DVLA: At-a-glance guide to the current medical standards of fitness to drive for medical practitioners available from 🖳 www.dvla.gov.uk

Medical advisers from the DVLA can advise on difficult issues – contact: Drivers Medical Unit, DVLA, Swansea SA99 1TU or ☎ 01792 761119

Drugs

British Society for Rheumatology: *National guidelines for the monitoring of second-line drugs* (2000) 🖳 www.rheumatology.org.uk

BNF 🖳 www.bnf.org

Obtaining steroid cards:
- England and Wales: Department of Health ☎ 08701 555 455
- Scotland: Banner Business Supplies ☎ 01506 448 440

HRT – see below

Falls in the elderly

Bandolier: *Falls in the elderly* –
🖳 www.jr2.ox.ac.uk/bandolier/band20/b20-5.html

Cochrane: Gillespie *et al. Interventions for preventing falls in elderly people.* (2002)

British Geriatric Society Falls and Bone Health Special Interest Group
🖳 www.falls-and-bone-health.org.uk

SIGN: *Prevention and management of hip fracture in older people* (2002)
🖳 www.sign.ac.uk

NICE: *Guidelines for the assessment and prevention of falls* (2004)
🖳 www.nice.org.uk

Feder *et al.* (2000) Guidelines for the prevention of falls in people over 65. *BMJ.* 321: 1007–11. 🖳 www.bmj.com

National Service Framework for Older People
🖳 www.dh.gov.uk

GP contract

DoH: *The GMS Contract* ▢ www.dh.gov.uk

BMA: *The Blue book and supporting documents*
▢ www.bma.org.uk

Head injury

NICE: *Triage, assessment investigation and early management of head injury in infants, children and adults* (2003) ▢ www.nice.org.uk

HRT

CSM Guidance: *Further advice on safety of HRT* (12/2003)
▢ www.mca.gov.uk

Million Women Study Collaborators. (2003) *Lancet*; 362: 419–27.

Women's Health Initiative Study ▢ www.whi.org

Industrial injury

RIDDOR: incident contact centre ☎ 0845 300 99 23
▢ www.riddor.gov.uk

Health and Safety Executive ☎ 0870 1545500
▢ www.hse.gov.uk

Jobcentre Plus ▢ www.jobcentreplus.gov.uk

Joint and soft tissue injection

Radcliffe Publishing Silver T. *Joint and soft tissue injection: injecting* with confidence (2001) ISBN: 1857755642

Osteoporosis

NICE ▢ www.nice.org.uk
- *Osteoporosis: secondary prevention* (2005)
- *Osteoporosis: assessment of fracture risk and prevention in high risk individuals* – due for publication in 2006.

National Osteoporosis Society: *Primary care strategy for osteoporosis and falls* (2002) ▢ www.nos.org.uk

Royal College of Physicians: *Osteoporosis: clinical guidelines for prevention and treatment* (2003) ▢ www.rcplondon.ac.uk

CSM Guidance: *Further advice on safety of HRT* (12/2003)
▢ www.mca.gov.uk

Pain

OUP: Moore *et al.* (2003), *Bandolier's little book of pain*,
ISBN: 0192632477

The Oxford Pain Internet Site
▢ www.jr2.ox.ac.uk/bandolier/booth/painpag

Polymyalgia rheumatica

Bird H.A. *et al.* (1979) An evaluation of criteria for polymyalgia rheumatica. *Annals of the rheumatic diseases.* 38(5): 434–9.

Sports medicine

British Association of Sport and Exercise Medicine
🖥 www.basem.co.uk

BMJ Publishing: *ABC of Sports Medicine* (1999) ISBN 072 791 3662

UK Sport: Drugs and sport card available from UK Sport,
40 Bernard Street, London WCA 1ST ☎ 020 7211 5100
🖥 www.uksport.gov.uk (Information resources)

Status of a particular medicine may be checked on the Drug Information Line ☎ 0800 528 0004 or 🖥 www.uksport.gov.uk/did

Information and contacts for patients, relatives and carers

General information
Arthritis Research Campaign (ARC) ☎ 0870 850 5000
🖳 www.arc.org.uk

Accidents
Royal Society for the Prevention of Accidents
🖳 www.rospa.co.uk

Ankylosing spondylitis
National Ankylosing Spondylitis Society (NASS) ☎ 01435 873527
🖳 www.nass.co.uk

Arthritis
Arthritis Research Campaign (ARC) ☎ 0870 850 5000
🖳 www.arc.org.uk

Arthritis Care ☎ 0808 800 4050 🖳 www.arthritiscare.org.uk

Arthritis Foundation 🖳 www.arthritis.org

Back pain
HMSO: *The back book* ISBN: 001 702 0788

Benefits
Benefit fraud line ☎ 0800 85 44 40

Citizens' Advice Bureau 🖳 www.adviceguide.org.uk

Department of Work and Pensions 🖳 www.dwp.gov.uk ☎ *Benefits Enquiry Line* – 0800 882200; 0800 243355 (minicom facility); 0800 441144 (for help with form completion)

Government information and services 🖳 www.direct.gov.uk

Inland Revenue 🖳 www.hmrc.gov.uk Tax credit enquiry line
☎ 0845 300 3900

Jobcentre Plus 🖳 www.jobcentreplus.gov.uk

Pension service 🖳 www.thepensionservice.gov.uk

Veterans Agency ☎ 0800 169 22 77
🖳 www.veteransagency.mod.uk

Brittle bones – see osteogenesis imperfecta

Carers

Carers UK ☎ 0808 808 7777 ⌨ www.carersonline.org.uk

Counsel and Care ☎ 0845 300 7585
⌨ www.counselandcare.org.uk

Princess Royal Trust for Carers ☎ 020 7480 7788
⌨ www.carers.org

Disability and carers' service ⌨ www.disability.gov.uk

Child abuse

Childline: 24-h. confidential counselling service ☎ 0800 1111
⌨ www.childline.org

Chronic fatigue syndrome

Action for ME ☎ 0845 123 2380 ⌨ www.afme.org.uk

ME Association ☎ 0870 444 1836 ⌨ www.meassociation.org.uk

Royal College of Psychiatrists: patient information sheets
⌨ www.rcpsych.ac.uk

Disability

Disabled Living Foundation ⌨ www.dlf.org.uk

Citizens' Advice Bureau ⌨ www.adviceguide.org.uk

Royal Association for Disability and Rehabilitation (RADAR) ☎ 020 7250
3222 ⌨ www.radar.org.uk

Disablement Information and Advice Line (DIAL) ☎ 01302 310123

Elderly

Age Concern ☎ 0800 00 99 66 ⌨ www.ageconcern.org.uk

Help the Aged ☎ 0800 800 65 65 ⌨ www.helptheaged.org.uk

Action on Elder Abuse ☎ 0808 808 8141 ⌨ www.elderabuse.org.uk

Falls

Royal Society for the Prevention of Accidents
⌨ www.rospa.co.uk

Fibromyalgia

Fibromyalgia Association UK ☎ 0870 220 1232
⌨ www.fibromyalgia-associationuk.org

STIFF(UK) ☎ 01782 562 366 ⌨ www.stiffuk.org

Foot problems

British Orthopaedic Foot Surgery Society
📟 www.bofss.org.uk

Hypermobility

Hypermobility Syndrome Association (HMSA)
📟 www.hypermobility.org

Lower limb problems

Steps ☎ 0871 717 0044 📟 www.steps-charity.org.uk

Lupus – see SLE

Osteogenesis imperfecta

Brittle Bone Society ☎ 08000 282 459 📟 www.brittlebone.org

Osteopetrosis

Osteopetrosis support trust 📟 www.ost.org.uk

Osteoporosis

National Osteoporosis Society ☎ 0845 450 0230
📟 www.nos.org.uk

Paget's disease

National Association for the Relief of Paget's Disease
☎ 0161 799 4646 📟 www.paget.org.uk

Psoriatic arthropathy

Psoriatic Arthropathy Alliance (PAA) ☎ 0870 770 3212
📟 www.paalliance.org

Raynaud's

Raynaud's and Scleroderma Association ☎ 01270 872776
📟 www.raynauds.org.uk

Restless legs

Restless Leg Syndrome Foundation 📟 www.rls.org

Ekbom Support Group 📟 www.ekbom.org.uk

Scleroderma

Raynaud's and Scleroderma Association ☎ 01270 872776
📟 www.raynauds.org.uk

Scoliosis

Scoliosis Association (UK) ☎ 020 8964 1166
📟 www.sauk.org.uk

Sjögren's syndrome

British Sjögren's Association ☎ 0121 455 6549
🖪 www.bssa.uk.net

SLE

Lupus UK ☎ 01708 731251 🖪 www.lupusuk.com

Spina bifida and hydrocephalus

Association for Spina Bifida and Hydrocephalus (ASBAH)
☎ 01733 555988 🖪 www.asbah.org.uk

Vasculitis

Stuart Strange Trust 🖪 www.vasculitis-uk.org

European Vasculitis Study Group 🖪 www.vasculitis.org

Kawasaki Support Group ☎ 024 7661 2178

Life support algorithms

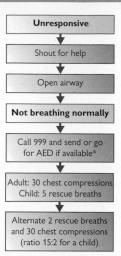

Basic life support (BLS) algorithm

Unresponsive

↓

Shout for help

↓

Open airway

↓

Not breathing normally

↓

Call 999 and send or go
for AED if available*

↓

Adult: 30 chest compressions
Child: 5 rescue breaths

↓

Alternate 2 rescue breaths
and 30 chest compressions
(ratio 15:2 for a child)

* For children, perform CPR for 1 minute before going for help

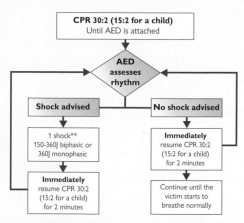

Automated external defibrillator (AED) algorithm

CPR 30:2 (15:2 for a child)
Until AED is attached

↓

**AED
assesses
rhythm**

Shock advised

↓

1 shock**
150-360J biphasic
or 360J monophasic

↓

Immediately
resume CPR 30:2
(15:2 for a child)
for 2 minutes

No shock advised

↓

Immediately
resume CPR 30:2
(15:2 for a child)
for 2 minutes

↓

Continue until the
victim starts to
breathe normally

** For children >8y. use adult AED. For children aged 1-8y. use paediatric pads
or paediatric mode if available else use as for adult. Not recommended for
children >1y.

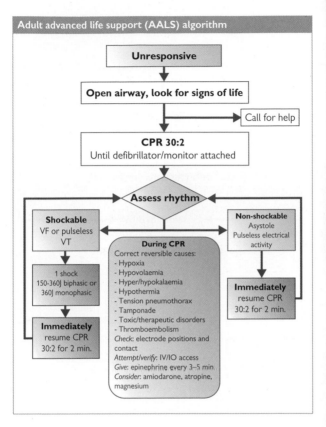

Adult advanced life support (AALS) algorithm

Unresponsive

Open airway, look for signs of life

Call for help

CPR 30:2
Until defibrillator/monitor attached

Assess rhythm

Shockable
VF or pulseless VT

1 shock
150-360J biphasic or 360J monophasic

Immediately
resume CPR 30:2 for 2 min.

During CPR
Correct reversible causes:
- Hypoxia
- Hypovolaemia
- Hyper/hypokalaemia
- Hypothermia
- Tension pneumothorax
- Tamponade
- Toxic/therapeutic disorders
- Thromboembolism
Check: electrode positions and contact
Attempt/verify: IV/IO access
Give: epinephrine every 3–5 min.
Consider: amiodarone, atropine, magnesium

Non-shockable
Asystole
Pulseless electrical activity

Immediately
resume CPR 30:2 for 2 min.

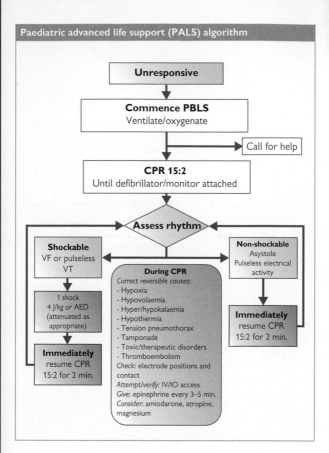

Paediatric advanced life support (PALS) algorithm

Unresponsive

↓

Commence PBLS
Ventilate/oxygenate

→ Call for help

↓

CPR 15:2
Until defibrillator/monitor attached

↓

Assess rhythm

Shockable
VF or pulseless VT

↓

1 shock
4 J/kg or AED
(attenuated as
appropriate)

↓

Immediately
resume CPR
15:2 for 2 min.

During CPR
Correct reversible causes:
- Hypoxia
- Hypovolaemia
- Hyper/hypokalaemia
- Hypothermia
- Tension pneumothorax
- Tamponade
- Toxic/therapeutic disorders
- Thromboembolism
Check: electrode positions and contact
Attempt/verify: IV/IO access
Give: epinephrine every 3–5 min.
Consider: amiodarone, atropine, magnesium

Non-shockable
Asystole
Pulseless electrical activity

↓

Immediately
resume CPR
15:2 for 2 min.

Index